Study Guide for Institutional Review Board: Management and Function
Second Edition

Amy L. Davis, JD, MPH

Elizabeth A. Bankert, MA

Karen Hansen

Susan Kornetsky, MPH, CIP

Helen McGough, MA, CIP

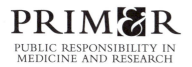

PRIM&R
PUBLIC RESPONSIBILITY IN
MEDICINE AND RESEARCH

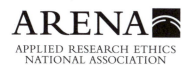

ARENA
APPLIED RESEARCH ETHICS
NATIONAL ASSOCIATION

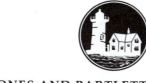

JONES AND BARTLETT PUBLISHERS
Sudbury, Massachusetts
BOSTON   TORONTO   LONDON   SINGAPORE

World Headquarters

Jones and Bartlett Publishers
40 Tall Pine Drive
Sudbury, MA 01776
978-443-5000
info@jbpub.com
www.jbpub.com

Jones and Bartlett Publishers
Canada
6339 Ormindale Way
Mississauga, Ontario L5V 1J2
Canada

Jones and Bartlett Publishers
International
Barb House, Barb Mews
London W6 7PA
United Kingdom

Jones and Bartlett books and products are available through most bookstores and online booksellers. To contact Jones and Bartlett Publishers directly, call 800-832-0034, fax 978-443-8000, or visit our website, www.jbpub.com.

Substantial discounts on bulk quantities of Jones and Bartlett publications are available to corporations, professional associations, and other qualified organizations. For details and specific discount information, contact the special sales department at Jones and Bartlett via the above contact information or send an e-mail to specialsales@jbpub.com.

The authors, editor, and publisher have made every effort to provide accurate information. However, they are not responsible for errors, omissions, or for any outcomes related to the use of the contents of this book and take no responsibility for the use of the products and procedures described. Treatments and side effects described in this book may not be applicable to all people; likewise, some people may require a dose or experience a side effect that is not described herein. Drugs and medical devices are discussed that may have limited availability controlled by the Food and Drug Administration (FDA) for use only in a research study or clinical trial. Research, clinical practice, and government regulations often change the accepted standard in this field. When consideration is being given to use of any drug in the clinical setting, the health care provider or reader is responsible for determining FDA status of the drug, reading the package insert, and reviewing prescribing information for the most up-to-date recommendations on dose, precautions, and contraindications, and determining the appropriate usage for the product. This is especially important in the case of drugs that are new or seldom used.

6048

Production Credits
Acquisitions Editor: Kevin Sullivan
Associate Editor: Amy Sibley
Editorial Assistant: Katilyn Crowley
Production Editor: Susan Schultz
Marketing Manager: Emily Ekle
Manufacturing and Inventory Coordinator: Amy Bacus
Text Design: Anne Spencer
Cover Design: Kristin E. Ohlin
Composition: Auburn Associates, Inc.
Printing and Binding: Malloy, Inc.

Printed in the United States of America
15 14 13 12 11   10 9 8 7 6 5 4 3

Contents

Preface

Public Responsibility in Research and Medicine (PRIM&R)/Applied Research Ethics National Association (ARENA) is pleased to publish this second edition of the study guide companion to the book *Institutional Review Board: Management and Function, Second Edition.* ARENA is the membership division of PRIM&R, a nonprofit organization dedicated to creating, implementing, and advancing the highest ethical standards in the conduct of research. PRIM&R/ARENA is the professional home for those whose responsibilities include the protection of human or animal research subjects. PRIM&R/ARENA's mission is to enhance human and animal research subject protections and the responsible conduct of research through the educational and professional development of its members. PRIM&R/ARENA's membership includes a range of professionals from research administrators, government officials, and academic deans to members and chairs of institutional review boards, institutional animal care and use committees, and institutional biosafety committees.

Over the past ten years there has been a "professionalization" of individuals who oversee and support institutional review board (IRB) functions. Ten years ago it was not uncommon for the secretary of the IRB chair to inherit the role of IRB administrator. The scope and complexity of clinical research have increased, as have the responsibilities assigned to individuals supporting IRBs and human subject protection programs. Those who perform leadership and oversight functions in human subject protection programs are under pressure to increase the sophistication and effectiveness of their operations. These demands require IRB administrators to obtain in-depth knowledge and continuing education in their field.

The textbook, *Institutional Review Board: Management and Function,* was the first book devoted to IRB administration. It was intended to be an instructional text focusing extensively on the procedures of IRB practice and the criteria for IRB decisions. Experts in the field of human subject protection wrote the individual chapters. After publication, PRIM&R/ARENA determined that there was a need for a companion study guide that could help individuals apply the knowledge they acquire from the textbook. An advisory group of PRIM&R/ARENA was formed to oversee the process of developing a study guide. Authors of *Institutional Review Board: Management and Function* were asked to develop study questions to emphasize key concepts in each of the chapters. These questions were carefully reviewed and edited by the advisory group. Once again, this study guide is written "by IRB people, for IRB people." Royalties from this study guide go directly to PRIM&R/ARENA to provide the organization with additional funds to continue to develop educational and networking programs.

Users should know a few important facts about the study guide before they begin to use it.

This study guide was written as a companion book to *Institutional Review Board: Management and Function, Second Edition.* Questions and answers are drawn directly from the text. Answer keys are included at the end of each section.

Some chapters represent an author's perspective of a particular issue or maybe even an example of a standard of practice for a particular institution. In these chapters, the questions and answers reflect the author's point of view, and other answers may also be appropriate. The editors have tried to make sure that there is only one correct answer to the question; however, the reader should keep in mind that the questions and answers directly correlate with the material in the chapter. The editors of this study guide do not assume responsibility for any wrong or incorrect information provided in the accompanying textbook.

As we are all aware, the field of human subject protection is not always black and white. There is ample room for interpretation. New regulations, policies, and guidelines emerge continually. Therefore, by the time this study guide goes to press, some of the topics covered in the text and the study guide may be out of date.

This book is not intended to be the sole resource for preparing for certification exams. This study guide may be one of many useful resources. Individuals preparing for a certification exam should review the resources recommended by the certification agencies.

We hope that this study guide will serve as a useful tool and will further the professional development of people working in the field of human subjects protection.

We welcome your comments on the study guide. Feedback on the value of this tool would be useful for consideration of future educational products of this kind. Please submit your comments to Amy Davis, either by e-mail at adavis@arena.org or by regular mail at Public Responsibility in Medicine and Research, 126 Brookline Avenue, Suite 202, Boston, MA 02215.

Amy Davis, JD, MPH
Elizabeth Bankert, MA
Karen Hansen
Susan Kornetsky, MPH, CIP
Helen McGough, MA, CIP

List of Contributors

Robert J. Amdur, MD
Elizabeth A. Bankert, MA
Deborah Barnard, MS, CIP
David A. Borasky, CIP
Timothy Callahan, PhD
Gary L. Chadwick, PharmD, MPH, CIP
Sanford Chodosh, MD
Jeffery M. Cohen, PhD
Jeffery A. Cooper, MD, MMM
Amy L. Davis, JD, MPH
Susan J. Delano, CIP
James M. Dubois, PhD, DSc
Michele Russell-Einhorn, JD
Kevin J. Epperson, CIP
Richard B. Ferrell, MD
Susan S. Fish, PharmD, MPH
David G. Forster, JD, MA, CIP
William L. Freeman, MD, MPH, CIP
Bruce G. Gordon, MD
Ronald M. Green, PhD
Bambi Grilley, RPh, CCRA, CCRC, CIP
Karen M. Hansen, BA
Erica J. Heath, MBA, CIP
Todd F. Heatherton, PhD
Rachel A. Hepp, BS, CIP
Kevin M. Hunt, CHFP
John M. Isidor, JD
Sandra P. Kaltman, RN, BSN, JD
Thomas G. Keens, MD
Felix Khin-Maung-Gyi, PharmD, MBA, CIP
Susan Z. Kornetsky, MPH, CIP
Gail Kotulak, BS

Christopher J. Kratochvil, MD
Robert J. Levine, MD
Sally L. Mann, MS, CIP
Peter Marshall, BA, CIP
Helen McGough, MA, CIP
Lawrence H. Muhlbaier, PhD
Daniel K. Nelson, MS, CIP
Robert M. Nelson, MD, PhD
Susan Nicholson, JD
J. Michael Oakes, PhD
Gwenn S.F. Oki, MPH
Tracy L. Ostler
Elisabeth A. Smith Parrott, CIP
Steven Peckman, MFA
Robin L. Penslar, JD
Ernest D. Prentice, PhD
Thomas Puglisi, PhD
Rebecca Carson Rogers, MA, CIP
Francine C. Romero, PhD, MPH
Patricia M. Scannell, CIP
Ada Sue Selwitz, MA
Laurie B. Slone, PhD
Marjorie A. Speers, PhD
Jennifer J. Tickle, PhD
Jan L. Trott, CIP
Pamela Wright, MA
Harold Y. Vanderpool, PhD, ThM
Daniel R. Vasgird, PhD, CIP
Cynthia S. Way, CIP, CCRP
Matthew D. Whalen, PhD
Mark R. Yessian, PhD

Acknowledgments

A very special thanks is given to the following individuals and organizations who supported this project and who strive to achieve excellence in the protection of human subjects:

Public Responsibility in Medicine and Research (PRIM&R)/Applied Research Ethics National Association (ARENA) for its financial and logistical support in the development of this study guide and for its role in fostering the professional growth of so many professionals working in the field of human subjects protection.

The individuals who volunteer to participate in research studies and who are essential partners in the effort to acquire new knowledge in behavioral, social, educational, and biomedical research.

The Study Guide Advisory Committee: Elizabeth Bankert, Karen Hansen, Susan Kornetsky, and Helen McGough, whose guidance and expertise ensure that this study guide is an effective educational resource for all human subject protection professionals.

Andie Hernandez, PRIM&R intern, for the many hours spent coordinating and copyediting this study guide.

Part 1

Background and Overview Topics

Chapter 1-1

An Ethics Primer for Institutional Review Boards

1. In this chapter, the author describes two major barriers that lead many institutional review boards (IRBs) to neglect to recognize and use ethical reasoning in their review of research protocols. He notes that the first of these barriers is erected by two sources: the Code of Federal Regulations (CFR) and *The Belmont Report*. Choose the answer that most accurately depicts the problem that the author describes with respect to these all-important documents for IRBs:

   a. Federal Regulations pay no attention to ethics, whereas *The Belmont Report* suggests that the Federal Regulations are seriously flawed.

   b. Neither the CFR nor *The Belmont Report* is truly applicable to modern medical research.

   c. The Federal Regulations do not emphasize the role of ethics and *The Belmont Report* does not explain how to use ethical reasoning to interpret and apply the regulations.

   d. *The Belmont Report* and the CFR contradict one another with respect to a number of issues that are important to IRB protocol review.

2. Choose the answer that most accurately describes what the author views as the second barrier to using ethical principles and reasoning in IRB deliberations:

   a. Many persons equate ethics with esoteric jargon and complex arguments rather than with principles and reasoning that are relied on in everyday life.

   b. Most of the time, people cannot agree on the ethical standards that apply to research involving human participants.

   c. IRB members do not spend enough time memorizing the Federal Regulations and reading *The Belmont Report*.

   d. IRB members do not appreciate the degrees to which actions that are not prohibited by federal regulations are ethical.

3. Choose the answer or answers that describe other major points emphasized in the author's chapter:

   a. In general, IRB's give far too much time and attention to the process of informed consent in their analysis of research protocols.

   b. IRB members should be required to take one or more courses—or at least one or more short courses—on research ethics.

   c. The "Applications" section of *The Belmont Report* is ethically stronger, more specific, and more applicable than its "Basic Ethical Principles" section.

   d. Ethical reasoning involves accurately determining the facts of the research in question, identifying the problem(s) posed by the research, and employing commonly used moral principles and arguments to arrive at the best ethical solution(s).

Chapter 1–2

Reflections of an Outsider

1. In June 1998 the U.S. Department of Health and Human Services Office of the Inspector General (OIG) issued a series of reports on IRBs. These reports list approximately six main deficiencies that threaten the effectiveness of the IRB system. Choose the answer that includes only those factors that were of major concern in the 1998 OIG reports:

   a. Excessive workload

      Minimal continuing review of approved research

      Lack of detail in informed consent documents

      Conflicts of interest that threaten independence

   b. Excessive workload

      Minimal continuing review of approved research

      Conflicts of interest that threaten independence

      Devoting little emphasis to the evaluation of IRB performance

   c. Providing little training to investigators or IRB members

      Outdated federal research regulations

      Conflicts of interest that threaten independence

      Devoting little emphasis to the evaluation of IRB performance

   d. Minimal continuing review of approved research

      Conflicts of interest that threaten independence

      Devoting little emphasis to the evaluation of IRB performance

      Excessive salaries for IRB staff

2. In this chapter, the author offers three main suggestions for protecting and improving the effectiveness of the IRB system. Choose the answer that lists the author's three main suggestions:

   a. Sustain a capacity for independent review, in substance and appearance.

      Strengthen continuing review.

      Require someone who is responsible for increasing research funding to serve on the IRB.

   b. Prohibit industry-sponsored research.

      Strengthen continuing review.

      Serve as an ambassador for human subjects' protection.

c. Sustain a capacity for independent review, in substance and appearance.

Focus more attention on the consent document.

Serve as an ambassador for human subjects' protection.

d. Sustain a capacity for independent review, in substance and appearance.

Strengthen continuing review.

Serve as an ambassador for human subjects' protection.

Chapter 1-3

A Unified Human-Research Protection Program

1. Public Responsibility in Medicine and Research (PRIM&R) was founded in 1974 with a mission to

   a. Develop a for-profit organization to educate institutions about IRB functions

   b. Lobby governmental agencies on issues concerning the protection of research subjects

   c. Promote the ethical conduct of human research through education of the scientific community and the public

   d. Supply regulatory agencies with consultants knowledgeable in human research

2. A well-integrated human research protection program should consist of

   a. An IRB consisting solely of knowledgeable scientists from within the institution

   b. An IRB consisting solely of nonscientists

   c. Policies and procedures relating to human research

   d. IRB members, IRB administrative staff, investigators, community and subject input, institutional oversight, and polices and procedures

3. The primary responsibility of the investigator is to the welfare of

   a. The institution

   b. The IRB

   c. Society

   d. The human subject in the investigation

4. Before the advent of federal regulations, the responsibility for the protection of human research subjects resided with

   a. The investigator

   b. The institution

   c. No specific individual or group

   d. Peer-review scientific journals

Chapter 1-4

A Shared Responsibility for Protecting Human Subjects

1. Choose the most accurate statement regarding a culture of respect for regulatory standards:

   a. A hostile relationship between the IRB and research community helps to support a culture of respect for the IRB within an organization.

   b. An IRB that spends most of its time polishing the wording in consent documents is likely to earn the respect of the research community.

   c. A culture of respect for the IRB will decrease research funding at an institution.

   d. A culture of respect for the IRB is difficult to regulate or standardize, yet it is more important than any other single consideration in protecting the rights and welfare of research subjects.

2. Choose the answer that most completely describes the components that make up the circle of trust:

   a. The investigator, the subject, and the investigator's boss

   b. The investigator, the subject, the federal government, the sponsoring institution, and the IRB

   c. The federal government, the subject, and the IRB

   d. The federal government, the IRB, and the investigator

Chapter 1-5

A Brief History of Public Responsibility in Medicine and Research and Institutional Review Board Education

1. The Mission of PRIM&R is to
   a. Lobby for regulations pertaining to IRBs
   b. Provide an educational forum for issues related to human subject research
   c. Provide consultants to IRBs
   d. Assist institutions in recruiting IRB members

2. In the 1970s the Presidential Commission contracted with PRIM&R to
   a. Organize an IRB conference
   b. Develop a guidebook for IRBs
   c. Commission a paper on informed consent
   d. Establish the first central IRB

3. The correct chronological order of Directors of the Office of Human Research protection is
   a. Chalkley, McCarthy, Ellis, and Koski
   b. McCarthy, Ellis, Chalkley, and Koski
   c. Ellis, Koski, McCarthy, and Chalkley
   d. McCarthy, Ellis, Koski, and Chalkley

Chapter 1-6

The Institutional Review Board: Definition and Federal Oversight

1. Choose the most accurate statement:

    a. Federal regulations require the Office for Human Research Protections (OHRP) to audit an IRB at least once a year.

    b. At an institution with an assurance of compliance with OHRP, research involving an investigational drug must be conducted in compliance with both HHS regulations at 45 CFR 46 and FDA regulations at 21 CFR 50 and 56.

    c. HHS and FDA regulations related to IRB review of research are identical in all respects.

    d. Federal law requires IRB approval for all research involving human subjects regardless of funding source or the nature of the research.

2. Choose the most accurate statement:

    a. Federal regulations require an OHRP investigation following the occurrence of an adverse event.

    b. Federal regulations require an FDA investigation following the publication of studies that describe noncompliant research practices.

    c. OHRP may restrict or suspend approval of an assurance for a research program that OHRP has determined does not operate in compliance with HHS regulations.

    d. Federal regulations require FDA audits every 4 years of research programs subject to FDA oversight.

Chapter 1-7

The Limits of Institutional Review Board Authority

1. Choose the answer that most accurately describes the message of this chapter:

   a. Federal regulations require the IRB to function as a Data and Safety Monitoring Board.

   b. Federal regulations require that the IRB regulate access to the results of genetic testing that is done for both research and nonresearch purposes.

   c. Federal regulations direct the IRB to function as a component of an organization's risk-management office.

   d. IRBs often find themselves in the position of being the most qualified or convenient group to do things that could be handled by another administrative body.

2. Which statement best characterizes the role of the IRB?

   a. The role of the IRB is to revise the consent document and develop procedures for protecting confidentiality of medical records.

   b. The role of the IRB is to protect the rights and welfare of human research participants by ensuring that the proposed informed consent process is appropriate and complete, that the procedures for protecting confidentiality are adequate, and that an appropriate system is in place to manage adverse events.

   c. The role of the IRB is to ensure that the research program is compliant with federal regulations and to identify practice patterns that might represent a legal liability for the institution.

   d. The role of the IRB is to ensure that research subjects receive adequate information about any additional costs that may result from participation in the research study.

ANSWER KEY FOR PART 1

Answer Key: Chapter 1-1

1. c
2. a
3. c and d

Answer Key: Chapter 1-2

1. b
2. d

Answer Key: Chapter 1-3

1. c
2. d
3. d
4. c

Answer Key: Chapter 1-4

1. d
2. b

Answer Key: Chapter 1-5

1. b
2. b
3. a

Answer Key: Chapter 1-6

1. b
2. c

Answer Key: Chapter 1-7

1. d
2. b

Part 2

Organizing the Office

Chapter 2-1

Administrative Reporting Structure for the Institutional Review Board

1. This chapter recommends that the best reporting structure for the institutional review board (IRB) is

   a. Specifically defined in the Department of Health and Human Services (DHHS) regulations at 45 CFR 46

   b. One that avoids a real or perceived conflict of interest

   c. One that reports to a faculty senate committee

   d. One that has a direct reporting relationship to the director of grants and contracts

2. This chapter recommends that the IRB chair report to

   a. The IRB office administrative staff

   b. The institutional official

   c. The executive committee of the medical staff

   d. The president of the faculty senate

3. Regardless of the size of an institution, its IRB should

   a. Be concerned with quality, efficiency, and consistency

   b. Have a minimum of three support staff

   c. Meet a minimum of twice a month

   d. Be concerned only with efficiency

4. The individual who signs the federalwide assurance on behalf of an institution is

   a. The director of grants and contracts

   b. The president of the faculty senate

   c. The institutional official

   d. The director of human resources

Chapter 2-2

Documentation, Policies, and Procedures

1. Federal regulations allow the IRB to invite individuals with competence in special areas to assist in the review of issues that require expertise beyond or in addition to that available on the IRB. When including such individuals (consultants) during the review

   a. The consultant counts toward quorum.

   b. The consultant may abstain from the vote.

   c. The consultant must leave the room after presenting the information requested by the IRB.

   d. The consultant may not vote.

2. The regulations found at 45 CFR 46.108 (a) require the IRB to follow written procedures for which of the following:

   a. Providing compensation to IRB members

   b. Providing education to investigators

   c. Reporting and reviewing adverse events

   d. Reporting unanticipated problems involving risks to subjects or others

3. The regulations define a quorum as

   a. One more than half of those present at the meeting

   b. One more than half of those present at the meeting and on the roster

   c. One more than half of those on the roster

   d. The regulations do not define quorum

4. When reviewing a study under the expedited review process, the reviewer may not

   a. Ask the investigator questions about the research proposal

   b. Request the investigator to make revisions to the research proposal

   c. Notify the investigator that the reviewer has disapproved the research

   d. Request the investigator to make revisions to the consent documents

Chapter 2-3

Tracking Systems Using Information Technology

1. According to the author, an electronic IRB allows an IRB to

    a. Establish more efficient business processes

    b. Maximize the use of available data

    c. Make consistent decisions that comply with regulations and institutional policies

    d. All of the above

2. According to the author, the most common reasons that IRBs seek information technology support is to

    a. Eliminate redundant data entry to better utilize staff and investigator time

    b. Eliminate printing and mailing documents resulting in conservation of human and material resources

    c. Reduce human errors to provide better quality data

    d. All of the above

3. The initial steps recommended by the author to develop an electronic system include

    a. An in-depth evaluation of the existing paper process and requirements for the e-submission system

    b. Development and analysis of a business process model and/or workflow diagram of areas that are to be automated and streamlined

    c. Identification and prioritization of essential development tasks

    d. All of the above

Chapter 2-4

Support Staff

1. Federal regulations on staffing the IRB office can be characterized as

   a. Very detailed and explicit

   b. Varied, depending entirely on which federal agency issued the regulations

   c. Implying only that an IRB be supported by an infrastructure

   d. Completely silent on the issue of staffing

2. Which of the following is NOT an IRB staff function?

   a. Preparation of the meeting agenda

   b. Prescreening proposals to be reviewed by the IRB

   c. Reviewing and approving proposed changes to approved projects

   d. Taking minutes at IRB meetings

3. Determining qualifications for IRB staff is

   a. Easy because there are degree programs in IRB management at most colleges and universities

   b. Easy because the tasks are primarily clerical

   c. Difficult because federal certification for staff members is required

   d. Difficult because of the wide variety and technical requirements of managing an IRB office

Chapter 2-5

Audit Systems

1. Which of the following statements reflects the requirements of DHHS regulations at 45 CFR 46?

    a. The IRB must audit the consent process.

    b. The IRB is not responsible for ensuring that there is adequate monitoring.

    c. Current interpretation of the regulations grant the institution, the IRB, and/or its representatives the authority to audit research.

    d. The IRB must perform semiannual audits of investigator records.

2. If evidence of serious or continuing noncompliance is found, which of the following statements is true in accordance with the requirements of DHHS regulations at 45 CFR 46.103(b)(5)?

    a. The noncompliance must only be reported to the IRB chair.

    b. The noncompliance must be immediately reported to the Office of Research Integrity (ORI).

    c. There are no specific follow-up requirements.

    d. The noncompliance must be reported promptly to the institutional official and the Office for Human Research Protections (OHRP).

3. Which of the following best characterizes a sound and effective research audit program?

    a. Audits should be proactive, nonpunitive, and focused on education.

    b. Audits should be conducted only for cause.

    c. Audits should be conducted objectively without dialog with the investigators.

    d. Audits should be conducted routinely without notice.

4. Major components of a successful research audit program include

    a. Endorsement and support of the audit program by senior institutional officials

    b. Adequate staffing by qualified individuals

    c. Quality control assessment and program improvement that are ongoing activities of the audit program itself

    d. All of the above

5. Which of the following criteria should be used for selecting the studies to be audited?

    a. Federally funded investigational new drug studies should be audited only if they are Phase I.

    b. Representative examples of all active studies should be audited.

    c. All commercially sponsored, investigational device exemption (IDE) studies should be audited.

    d. Only studies that have enrolled at least 100 subjects should be audited.

Chapter 2-6

Charging for Institutional Review Board Review

1. Which of the following statements concerning charging a fee for IRB review is correct?

   a. Review fees are prohibited by the DHHS regulations at 45 CFR 46.

   b. Pharmaceutical companies do not object to paying reasonable IRB review fees.

   c. The entire IRB operation budget should come from review fees.

   d. The IRB review fee should be charged only if the study is approved.

2. Which of the following statements concerning charging for IRB review is correct?

   a. Resources currently are not a problem in today's culture of compliance.

   b. Support for the IRB should come primarily from the institution.

   c. IRB review fees should be increased slowly in order to replace institutional support.

   d. IRB review fees are a detriment to an investigator's ability to obtain contracts.

ANSWER KEY FOR PART 2

Answer Key: Chapter 2-1

1. b
2. b
3. a
4. c

Answer Key: Chapter 2-2

1. d
2. d
3. d
4. c

Answer Key: Chapter 2-3

1. d
2. d
3. d

Answer Key: Chapter 2-4

1. c
2. c
3. d

Answer Key: Chapter 2-5

1. c
2. d
3. a
4. d
5. b

Answer Key: Chapter 2-6

1. b
2. b

Part 3

Organizing the Institutional Review Board Committee

Chapter 3-1

Reflections on Chairing an Institutional Review Board

1. In this chapter, the author presents six recommendations on which institutional review board (IRB) chairs should focus to improve IRB function. These recommendations are equally applicable to IRB administrative directors and others in a position of leadership related to research regulation. Choose the answer that includes three of the author's recommendations:

   a. Attempt to solve problems when they are small.

   Establish an adversarial relationship between the IRB and researchers.

   Make a commitment to continuing education.

   b. Assemble the right team.

   Treat researchers as trusted colleagues.

   Explain to researchers that many IRB policies exist mainly to satisfy the "Feds."

   c. Attempt to solve problems when they are small.

   Treat researchers as trusted colleagues.

   Make a commitment to continuing education.

   d. Take a retroactive rather than a proactive approach to problem management.

   Treat researchers as trusted colleagues.

   Make a commitment to continuing education.

Chapter 3-2

The Institutional Review Board Chair

1. Which of the following best describes the responsibilities of an IRB chair who plans to function as a comprehensive IRB professional?

    a. To play a leadership role in establishing and implementing IRB policy, represent the IRB in discussions with federal authorities and other segments of the organization, and participate fully as an IRB member

    b. To promote the concept that the IRB is not an administrative obstacle to conducting research

    c. To promote an adversarial relationship between the researchers and the IRB

    d. To require an IRB member other than the chair to defend IRB decisions to researchers

2. Which of the following sets of skills and characteristics are most essential for a well-qualified IRB chair who plans to function as a comprehensive IRB professional?

    a. Ability to foster open and collaborative discussion at the full-committee IRB meeting

    b. Supervise other IRB members in discussing IRB concerns with investigators

    c. Possess a medical degree

    d. Be actively involved in the majority of protocols of the local research community

3. Choose the answer that best describes the recommended time commitment required to chair an IRB that conducts full-committee review of approximately 200 new protocols per year:

    a. The time it takes each month to conduct the full-committee meeting(s)

    b. Approximately 40 hours each week

    c. Approximately 15–30% of a full-time equivalent position

    d. One hour per week in addition to full-committee meetings

Chapter 3-3

The Institutional Review Board Administrative Director

1. Choose the statement that most accurately reflects the information presented in this chapter:

   a. It is never appropriate for the IRB administrative director to represent the organization in discussion with federal authorities or to triage research between IRB review categories.

   b. The authors recommend that the IRB administrative director's responsibilities be limited to that of an administrator who is responsible only for procedural aspects of the IRB meeting.

   c. The authors strongly recommend that the IRB administrative director be an expert on policy and regulations that relate to the details of IRB function.

   d. The IRB administrative director should require that the organization hire an attorney to advise the IRB on the interpretation of federal research regulations.

2. Choose the statement that most accurately reflects the information presented in this chapter:

   a. An effective IRB should not have a collegial relationship with members of the research community.

   b. The IRB office should function as a "research service center" that actively assists the researcher in going through the IRB review process.

   c. IRB administrative staff should not participate in helping researchers write the consent document.

   d. Federal regulations require that the IRB administrative director be a member of the IRB committee.

3. Choose the statement that most accurately reflects the information presented in this chapter:

   a. The IRB administrative director may approve research by the expedited procedure so long as he or she has been authorized to perform this function by the IRB chair, is an experienced IRB reviewer, and is a current member of the IRB committee.

   b. Federal regulations require the IRB administrative director to organize educational programs for IRB members.

   c. The IRB administrative director should have sole responsibility for determining when new research should be considered exempt from further IRB review.

   d. Federal regulations require the administrative director to advise other institutional departments on issues related to privacy and confidentiality of health information.

Chapter 3-4

The Role of an Attorney

1. This chapter discusses three models for attorney participation on an IRB. Which model would not be appropriate for an attorney serving on an IRB?

   a. Assists/guides the IRB in a manner that helps them analyze a circumstance

   b. Reviews the IRB action after the IRB meeting and provides feedback to the chairperson

   c. Advises the IRB on the pertinent federal, state, and local regulations

   d. Advises the committee on ancillary legal matters

2. The author states that an IRB that lacks an attorney member:

   a. Is out of compliance with federal regulations

   b. Is not permitted to review biomedical research

   c. Must have a paralegal as a substitute

   d. Is permitted within the regulations, but not advised

3. According to this author, an attorney who is a voting member of the IRB should NOT provide advice on which of the following topics:

   a. The definition of mature minors and emancipated minors

   b. The definition of legally authorized representatives

   c. The interpretation of the Health Insurance Portability and Accountability Act (HIPAA)

   d. Steps to be taken to protect the institution

4. Which of the following statements is correct?

   a. An attorney on an IRB must also be the in-house counsel of the institution.

   b. An IRB must have both an in-house and external attorney.

   c. Only an attorney from outside the institution should sit on an IRB.

   d. Whether an external or internal attorney sits on an IRB may depend on the role he or she is expected to fulfill.

Chapter 3-5

Committee Size, Alternates, and Consultants

1. Choose the answer in which all statements correctly reflect Department of Health and Human Services (DHHS) and Food and Drug Administration (FDA) regulatory requirements concerning the size and composition of the IRB:

   a. Each IRB must have at least seven members.

      At least one IRB member must be a scientist who is not affiliated with the IRB's institution.

      Each IRB must have an expert in research involving vulnerable populations.

   b. Each IRB must have at least five members.

      At least one IRB member must be a scientist.

      Half of the IRB members must be closely associated with the IRB's institution.

   c. Each IRB must have at least five members.

      At least one IRB member must be a scientist.

      At least half of the IRB members must be nonscientists.

   d. At least one IRB member must be a scientist.

      At least one IRB member must be a nonscientist.

      At least one IRB member must have no meaningful association with the IRB's institution.

2. Choose the most accurate statement regarding IRB membership:

   a. The number of members who must be present to make quorum for a full-committee meeting is lower for an IRB with eight member positions than for an IRB with nine member positions.

   b. Input from an appropriately qualified consultant may be a useful way to supplement IRB expertise.

   c. An "alternate" IRB member may serve as a voting member at a full-committee meeting without prior approval from the Office for Human Research Protections as long as it is documented that the regular IRB member is not able to attend the meeting.

   d. Appointing an "alternate member-at-large" to the IRB increases the number of members required for a full-committee quorum.

3. Choose the most accurate statement regarding the size of the IRB.

   a. Federal regulations require that the number of IRB members be proportionate to the volume and complexity of the studies that the IRB reviews.

   b. Administrative costs associated with IRB operations should determine the size of the IRB.

   c. The size of the IRB should allow members to feel comfortable engaging in open discussion, asking questions, and disagreeing with each other.

   d. Large IRBs are recommended for ease of achieving a quorum.

Chapter 3-6

Length, Frequency, and Time of Institutional Review Board Meetings

1. Choose the answer that includes three factors that are likely to determine the optimal length, time, and frequency of IRB full-committee meetings:

   a. Administrative efficiency

      Federal regulations that require at least two nonscientists to hold a meeting

      Volume of items that require full-committee review

   b. Volume of items that require full-committee review

      Member availability

      State law

   c. Member availability

      Ability to maintain a quorum

      Federal regulations require meetings at least once a month

   d. Volume of items that require full-committee review

      Member availability

      Administrative efficiency

Chapter 3-7

Institutional Review Board Subcommittees

1. DHHS regulations at 45 CFR 46.110 describe the requirements for IRB review of research using an expedited process. Choose the answer that summarizes an activity that would violate these regulatory requirements:

   a. Expedited review of research by a single person who is an experienced IRB member and designated to perform this task by the IRB chair

   b. Expedited review of research by the IRB administrative director for an IRB where the administrative director is not a voting member of the IRB committee

   c. Expedited review of research by a subcommittee consisting of three experienced IRB members who are designated to perform this task by the IRB chair

   d. Research that does not meet standards for approval by an expedited process and is referred to the full IRB committee for review

2. Choose the answer that best describes a situation or situations in which the use of an IRB subcommittee is permitted by federal regulations and likely to improve the efficiency and quality of IRB function:

   a. To approve research that is high risk in a situation where the potential benefit of the research will be lost if research is delayed until the next full-committee IRB meeting

   b. To disapprove a research application that is unlikely to be approved by the full committee

   c. To eliminate the need for all IRB members to consider the substantive issues in a protocol that requires full-committee review

   d. To review research by an expedited process, to review requests for minor revisions to approved research, and/or to conduct compliance audits

3. Choose the answer that best describes the process recommended by the authors for reviewing Serious Adverse Event Reports (SAERs):

   a. All SAERs should be reviewed first by the IRB chair and then by the full committee.

   b. All SAERs should be reviewed first by the investigator who provides his or her assessment to the IRB chair. The IRB chair then determines whether the occurrence of the adverse event changes the risk to research subjects, in which case he or she forwards the AER for full-committee review.

   c. All SAERs should be reviewed first by a qualified subcommittee, which makes a determination of whether the adverse event suggests a change in the risk to research subjects in which case the subcommittee forwards the AER for full-committee review.

   d. All SAERs should be reviewed by the investigator who determines whether the study should be suspended.

Chapter 3-8

Social Science vs. Biomedical Institutional Review Boards

1. Choose the most accurate statement:

   a. Federal regulations hold social science and biomedical research to different standards.

   b. Social harms are real harms that may compromise the quality of life of research participants as much as serious physical harm.

   c. Social harm is important to consider during IRB review of social science research, but social harm does not occur with biomedical research.

   d. Federal regulations prohibit a single IRB from reviewing both social science and biomedical research studies.

2. Choose the most accurate statement:

   a. Both biomedical and social research involves risks of social and physical harm.

   b. When the workload is too heavy for one IRB, it is recommended that the work be segregated between two or more IRBs based on whether the research is social science or biomedical.

   c. Social harms that may occur as a result of participation in biomedical or social science research include loss of employability, loss of insurability, embarrassment, and discrimination.

   d. Separate IRB review of social science and biomedical research is recommended to increase the effectiveness of IRB review.

ANSWER KEY FOR PART 3

Answer Key: Chapter 3-1

1.   c

Answer Key: Chapter 3-2

1.   a
2.   a
3.   c

Answer Key: Chapter 3-3

1.   c
2.   b
3.   a

Answer Key: Chapter 3-4

1.   b
2.   d
3.   d
4.   d

Answer Key: Chapter 3-5

1.   d
2.   b
3.   c

Answer Key: Chapter 3-6

1.   d

Answer Key: Chapter 3-7

1.   b
2.   d
3.   b

Answer Key: Chapter 3-8

1.   b
2.   c

Part 4

Review Categories

Chapter 4-1

Exempt from Institutional Review Board Review

1. Which of the following best describes the party(s) responsible for determining whether a research study meets the criteria for exemption:

   a. An investigator

   b. An institutional review board (IRB) office staff person who is not a member of the IRB

   c. A research study nurse

   d. A research study coordinator

2. Exempt research can never involve which of the following classes of subjects?

   a. Pregnant women

   b. Decisionally impaired, homeless individuals

   c. Prisoners

   d. Nursing home residents

3. Which of the following statements best describes exempt research:

   a. It is exempt from compliance with DHHS regulations at 45 CFR 46.

   b. It requires continuation reports and reports of the occurrence of unanticipated problems.

   c. It is exempt from compliance with the Health Insurance Portability and Accountability Act (HIPPA) Privacy Rule.

   d. It is exempt from compliance with the FDA regulations.

Chapter 4-2

Expedited Institutional Review Board Review

1. In accordance with Department of Health and Human Services (DHHS) and Food and Drug Administration (FDA) regulatory requirements, expedited review can be conducted on

    a. Amendments, such as adding a placebo arm to a study that was previously reviewed and approved at a convened meeting of the IRB

    b. A study involving no more than minimal risk and one that is on the DHHS- and FDA-specified list of categories eligible for expedited review

    c. Clinical studies that involve more than minimal risk for which the institution's IRB has had a lot of experience reviewing

    d. Continuation reports for studies that involve more than minimal risk but for which only one subject has been entered during the reporting period

2. In accordance with DHHS regulation, who can conduct expedited review?

    a. The IRB office staff who are not voting members of the IRB but who have a lot of IRB and research experience

    b. A faculty member who is not an IRB member but who has demonstrated expertise in the research being reviewed

    c. The IRB chair, other IRB members designated by the chair, or a subcommittee of the IRB

    d. The department chair of the study investigator

3. Minor modifications of a currently approved protocol can be reviewed by expedited process. Choose the answer that reflects the best example of a minor modification:

    a. Temporary closure of a study due to recent adverse events and the need to analyze data before further subject accrual can resume

    b. Changes in study entry criteria

    c. Substitution of one drug for a different drug

    d. Changes to the principal investigator's telephone number on the consent form

4. When conducting expedited review, the authorized reviewer must do the following:

    a. Determine that the study meets the same criteria for approval as a study that may be reviewed by the full board

    b. Determine that the study is not a replication study

    c. Determine that the study cannot be approved and send a letter to the investigator informing him or her that the study has been disapproved

    d. Disapprove the study and inform the IRB of this determination at the next meeting

5. Choose the answer that reflects a pediatric study that can be reviewed by expedited review:

   a. Venipuncture in normal, healthy infants

   b. Skin biopsy in children with hemophilia

   c. Bone marrow biopsy in children with leukemia

   d. Venipuncture in children with needle phobia

6. Continuing review of research previously approved by a convened IRB can be reviewed by the expedited review process when

   a. All subjects have expired and the study will end 2 months after IRB approval has expired.

   b. No subjects have been enrolled and no additional risks have been identified in a gene transfer study.

   c. No new subjects will be enrolled and two subjects are still on active treatment.

   d. No subjects have been enrolled and a recent report indicates that subjects on another study using the same drug experienced a grade 4 unexpected adverse event.

Chapter 4-3

Identifying Intent: Is This Project Research?

1. Choose the answer that best describes three activities that appropriately may be classified as something other than research:

   a. Nonvalidated medical practice

      Public health interventions

      Quality assessment/improvement

   b. Phase I testing of investigational medications

      Medical practice for the benefit of others

      Resource utilization review

   c. Off-label use of approved medications

      Randomized clinical trials

      Quality improvement

   d. Quality assessment

      Nonvalidated medical practice

      Placebo-controlled trials

2. Choose the answer that best describes a defining characteristic of research, according to the authors:

   a. A systematic investigation that may invade the privacy of medical patients

   b. A systematic investigation that involves interventions that are designed solely to enhance the well-being of an individual patient

   c. Publication of results in an academic journal

   d. A major goal of the activity is to learn something for the purpose of benefiting people other than the research subjects

3. Choose the most accurate statement:

   a. Quality Improvement projects are aimed at improving medical systems nationwide.

   b. HIPAA allows a covered entity to obtain information related to treatment, payment, or health care operations without additional patient consent.

   c. A case report constitutes a systematic investigation such that it would always be considered "research" under the federal regulations.

   d. Innovative therapy is always considered "research" within the meaning of the federal regulations.

4. Choose the answer that most accurately describes the question that the authors use to identify research intent:

   a. Is there any chance that the results of this project will be submitted for publication in an academic journal?

   b. Is any type of innovative therapy or testing being used in this project?

   c. Would the project be conducted as planned if the project director knew he or she would never receive any form of academic recognition for it?

   d. Is the project director on faculty at an academic institution that conducts research?

Chapter 4-4

Compassionate Use and Emergency Use Exemption

1. Choose the most accurate statement:

   a. The 1993 Office for Protection from Research Risks (OPRR) *IRB Guidebook* discourages use of the term *compassionate use* because it may confuse discussions about the need for IRB approval of research.

   b. Federal regulations permit IRBs to approve the use of investigational medications on a "compassionate-use" basis outside the setting of a formal research protocol.

   c. Federal regulations permit the IRB chair to give IRB approval for the use of an investigational drug without a full committee meeting as long as the drug is being used on a "compassionate-use" basis.

   d. Federal regulations specify that "compassionate-use" protocols are exempt from IRB review.

2. Choose the most accurate statement:

   a. According to FDA regulations, an investigational medication may be used without IRB approval whenever it is likely to benefit a patient in a meaningful way.

   b. According to FDA regulations, the study sponsor and local investigator do not need prior IRB approval to use an investigational medication in a situation that meets the FDA definition of "emergency use."

   c. DHHS regulations at 45 CFR 46 permit the conduct of research without IRB approval in an "emergency-use" situation.

   d. FDA regulations permit the use of an investigational medication on a "compassionate use" basis without full-committee IRB approval as long as no more than five subjects are treated.

3. Choose the most accurate statement:

   a. FDA regulations require IRB approval to use an investigational medication in an "emergency-use" situation.

   b. When notified of the use of an investigational medication without prior IRB approval in an "emergency-use" situation, the IRB chair or administrative director should generate a letter stating that the IRB approves of the situation.

   c. FDA regulations require a local investigator/physician to notify the IRB within 5 days of the use of an investigational medication without IRB approval in an "emergency-use" situation.

   d. DHHS regulations at 45 CFR 46 permit a local investigator to administer an investigational medication for research purposes in an "emergency-use" situation without IRB approval.

4. Choose the most accurate statement to complete the following sentence: An investigator who requests emergency use of an FDA-regulated drug, biologic, or device that is the subject of research funded by DHHS and FDA

   a. Must seek IRB approval because the patient is considered a research participant

   b. Must follow FDA regulations and request an acknowledgment letter from the IRB

   c. Must request an acknowledgment letter from the IRB and may not use the resulting data as part of a prospective research study

   d. Would be denied

Chapter 4-5

Waiver of Consent in Emergency Medicine Research

1. Informed consent may be completely waived in emergency medicine research when

    a. The research involves an investigational intervention under FDA special regulation at 21 CFR 50.24

    b. Any unconscious patient requires emergency medical care

    c. The research is to be conducted with minors, pregnant women, or prisoners

    d. The researcher does not have the personnel available to obtain consent

2. A researcher approaches the IRB to request a waiver of consent to administer an investigational drug to people who have suffered a stroke and are brought to the hospital by ambulance. Which of the following questions should the IRB ask the researcher in relation to the waiver request? (Answer Yes or No for each of the following.)

    a. Will the data collected from the subjects be published?

    b. Has the researcher filed a special IND with the FDA?

    c. Has the researcher obtained permission from the subjects' primary care providers before entering them into the research protocol?

    d. Has the researcher developed a procedure for informing subjects about their participation at the first available opportunity?

    e. Has the community voted to approve or disapprove the research?

3. Who is responsible for public notification and community consultation when it is anticipated that a waiver of consent in emergency medicine research will be required?

    a. The sponsor of the study

    b. The researcher

    c. The IRB

    d. The regulations do not specify who is to do this

4. Despite the fact that the regulations allow a waiver of consent in emergency medicine research, the regulations also require that some consenting procedures be followed. Which of the following must be developed before the waiver can be approved? (Answer Yes or No for each of the following.)

    a. A written consent form to be signed by the subject's legally authorized representative before the subject can be enrolled.

    b. Consent from the subject as soon as he or she becomes competent to provide it.

    c. A procedure for identifying the subject's legally authorized representative.

    d. A protocol for contacting a subject's family members when it is not possible to contact the subject's legally authorized representative.

5. If an IRB does not approve a study involving waiver of consent in emergency medicine research, which of the following actions are required by the regulations?

    a. Suspend the researcher from submitting future projects to the IRB.

    b. Notify the other IRBs that have reviewed the study of its determination.

    c. Notify the community that it has not approved the study.

    d. Require that the study be conducted without a waiver of informed consent.

6. What special regulatory membership requirements are there for an IRB that reviews requests for waivers of consent in emergency medicine research?

    a. No special requirement

    b. A specialist in emergency medicine

    c. A representative from the target community

    d. Legal counsel

ANSWER KEY FOR PART 4

Answer Key: Chapter 4-1

1. b
2. c
3. a

Answer Key: Chapter 4-2

1. b
2. c
3. d
4. a
5. a
6. b

Answer Key: Chapter 4-3

1. a
2. d
3. b
4. c

Answer Key: Chapter 4-4

1. a
2. b
3. c
4. c

Answer Key: Chapter 4-5

1. a
2. a, yes

    b, yes

    c, no

    d, yes

    e, no
3. d
4. a, no

    b, no

    c, yes

    d, yes
5. b
6. a

Part 5

Initial Protocol Review and the Full-Committee Meeting

Chapter 5-1

Overview of Initial Protocol Review

1. *At the very least*, the _____ signature should be obtained on a protocol application, to indicate that this person _____.

   a. Investigator's; takes full responsibility for the conduct of the research and conformance with human subject protections

   b. Investigator's; will report any noncompliance to the Office for Human Research Protections (OHRP)

   c. Hospital president's; will pay for the entire research study

   d. Hospital president's; will obtain informed consent

2. The purpose of the institutional review board (IRB) Reviewer Worksheet is to

   a. Help promote consistent and thorough review by IRB members

   b. Document that IRB review occurred

   c. Help the IRB comply with Department of Health and Human Services (DHHS) and Food and Drug Administration (FDA) regulations

   d. Educate IRB members about the IRB review process

   e. All of the above

3. The following statement supports which one of the criteria for IRB approval of research?

   "*Blood for research lab tests will be drawn at the same time as for clinically indicated labs so that an extra needle stick is not necessary.*"

   a. Informed consent will be appropriately documented.

   b. Risks to subjects are reasonable in relationship to anticipated benefits.

   c. Risks to subjects are minimized.

   d. Subject selection is equitable.

4. Which one of the following statements is true?

   a. IRBs are required to have submission deadlines and meet on a monthly basis.

   b. IRBs are required to conduct continuing review at intervals appropriate to the degree of risk for each study and, *at a minimum*, annually.

   c. IRBs do not have to review the informed consent documents being used in a study, as this is the investigator's responsibility.

   d. IRBs are not required to evaluate the scientific justification of a study.

Chapter 5-2

Evaluating Study Design and Quality

1. Choose the most accurate statement regarding IRB review of study design and other factors that determine the quality of the science in a research project:

    a. The IRB has no business evaluating study design in a research project.

    b. Federal regulations do not mention study design as a criterion for IRB approval of research.

    c. An IRB that functions in compliance with federal regulations and accepted ethical codes has an obligation to evaluate study design and other factors that affect risk and benefits.

    d. The IRB should not question the study design in projects that involve a medication that has been given an investigational new drug number by the FDA.

2. Choose the most accurate statement about a study that is so poorly designed that it is unlikely to yield persuasive results regarding the study hypothesis:

    a. Federal regulations direct the IRB to approve the study as long as the risk to subjects is low.

    b. The IRB should consider only the importance of the research question, not the chance that the study will generate meaningful results.

    c. The study probably violates the Nuremberg Code and federal regulations at 45 CFR 46.111(a)(1).

    d. Poor quality research is always better than no research.

3. For IRBs, which are called on to evaluate the scientific issues for a wide range of protocols requiring different areas of expertise beyond those of its membership, the best practice is to

    a. Hire consultants having the relevant expertise for each scientific inquiry necessary.

    b. Establish new IRBs having different areas of expertise.

    c. Focus on the ethics rather than the science.

    d. Establish a scientific review system that occurs before IRB review.

Chapter 5-3

The Study Population: Women, Minorities, and Children

1. The regulation requiring equitable selection of research subjects is based on which of the following principles:

    a. Research involving human subjects should be conducted only if the importance of the objective outweighs the inherent risks and burdens to the subject.

    b. Research subjects should be treated as autonomous agents.

    c. The burdens and benefits of research must be fairly distributed.

    d. Recruitment procedures may not be coercive or misleading.

2. A protocol is presented to the IRB that proposes to study the effectiveness of a drug to treat hypertension. The recruitment plan is to enroll both men and women between the ages of 40 and 65. Which of the following best describes the information required by the IRB to assess the ethics of the recruitment plan?

    a. Data from prior studies that demonstrate the effect of the drug on animal subjects

    b. Whether the protocol includes a placebo arm

    c. Whether the risks of participating in the study outweigh the benefits to society

    d. Whether prior studies demonstrate that men and women are diagnosed with hypertension at comparable rates at comparable ages

3. To exclude a particular subject population in an FDA-regulated drug study, the IRB must

    a. Consider the rationale for exclusion criteria

    b. Accept the sponsor's eligibility criteria

    c. Accept the criteria because FDA-approved the investigational new drug (IND) process

    d. Consider the economic burden on the investigator to do equitable recruitment

4. A research study of a drug to treat cholesterol excludes pregnant women from the study. The researchers have incorporated this exclusion criterion into the protocol to protect the fetus from unknown harms that might be associated with the study drug. This exclusion criterion is reasonable because

    a. There is significant risk of harm from the drug to a fetus.

    b. It is equitable to subject a potential fetus to the same risk to which an adult female would be subjected.

    c. Women are likely at lower risk than men of developing heart disease from elevated cholesterol levels.

    d. Protecting the health of a fetus from the unknown harms that might be associated with the study drug is a clear and compelling reason to exclude pregnant women from the study population.

Chapter 5-4

Community Consultation to Assess and Minimize Group Harms

1. Which of the following procedures will hinder IRB consideration of the risk of group harms?

    a. Including members on the IRB who are members of the group to be studied

    b. Consulting with members of the population to be studied

    c. Consulting only with the researcher about the possibility of group harms

    d. Consulting with IRBs with previous experience with the subject population to be studied

2. Jurisdiction by tribal governments over the conduct of research extends to

    a. All research with Native American peoples, even research not conducted on a reservation

    b. All research conducted on reservations

    c. All research except that conducted by the U.S. Indian Health Service

    d. No research—tribal governments do not have jurisdiction in this area

3. Which of the following is NOT a valid reason for IRBs to ask principal investigators of nonemergency research involving a distinct minority or vulnerable group to consult with the community?

    a. To identify potential harms that the researcher and IRB are not aware of

    b. To identify potential benefits that the researcher and IRB are not aware of

    c. To comply with federal regulations requiring community consultation in such circumstances

    d. To understand better the setting, leading to better research methods

4. Which of the following does NOT describe a type or types of group risks identified by the authors.

    a. Internal and external genetic determinism and stigmatization

    b. Disruption of the tribe's values

    c. Increase distrust of the health care system

    d. Risk to employment status

Chapter 5-5

Privacy and Confidentiality

1. DHHS and FDA regulations require that the IRB determine for each protocol that there are adequate provisions to protect the privacy of subjects and maintain the confidentiality of data. Choose the answer that portrays the provision to provide sufficient information for the IRB to make its required determination:

   a. The study records are kept in a locked file cabinet in the investigator's office.

   b. The study records are kept on a computer with password protection.

   c. The study records are kept in the investigator's office; those records use a coded identification number to identify each subject, and the list that provides links between the coded identification numbers and the subjects' identities is stored separately in a locked file cabinet in the investigator's office.

   d. The study records are kept in the investigator's academic department.

2. Choose the most accurate statement regarding subject confidentiality and privacy during subject recruitment activities:

   a. Recruitment activities do not involve issues of confidentiality and privacy.

   b. The collection of information during recruitment activities may require careful consideration of confidentiality and privacy.

   c. The federal regulations state that IRBs do not have to review recruitment activities.

   d. Confidentiality and privacy are only concerns during recruitment into federally funded research studies.

3. Which one of the following federal agencies has issued guidance stating that research subjects should be informed in the consent form that the agency may review the subjects' individual medical records?

   a. The National Institutes of Health

   b. The Federal Bureau of Investigation

   c. The Food and Drug Administration

   d. The Department of Education

4. When an IRB reviews research involving the collection of information from a research subject about the family members of that subject, what issue will the IRB likely have to consider based on privacy concerns and the definition of "human subject" in the Common Rule?

   a. Secondary subjects

   b. Adequate birth control

   c. Consent for autopsies

   d. Compensation for injury

5. Which of the two following *Belmont* principles most directly support the need for maintaining confidentiality and privacy in research?

   a. Justice and respect for persons

   b. Justice and beneficence

   c. Respect for persons and beneficence

   d. Respect for persons and charity

6. How does the International Conference on Harmonisation (ICH) differ from the FDA regulations and the Common Rule regarding the information about confidentiality that must be included in the consent form?

   a. The ICH explicitly requires that subjects be informed that various individuals might review their original medical records, including monitors, auditors, the IRB, and government authorities, whereas the FDA regulations and the Common Rule are not as explicit.

   b. The ICH defers to local law on this issue, whereas the FDA regulations and the Common Rule set a higher standard.

   c. The ICH, the FDA regulations, and the Common Rule are identical.

   d. The ICH requires only a statement that there are policies in place to protect confidentiality, whereas the FDA regulations and the Common Rule use the opposite approach and require that there be a list of people provided in the consent form who will have access to the study data.

Chapter 5-6

Recruitment of Research Subjects

1. The beginning of the informed consent process is when a potential subject

    a. First becomes aware of the clinical trial

    b. Sets an appointment with the investigator/study coordinator to discuss possible participation

    c. Reads the informed consent

    d. Signs the informed consent

2. The Office of the Inspector General Report on "Recruiting Human Subjects: Pressures in Industry-Sponsored Clinical Research" of 2000 is still relevant because

    a. The report constitutes formal guidance.

    b. There have been no significant developments since.

    c. The report states that reviewing recruitment methods provides additional opportunity for oversight bodies to monitor the actual content of the consent process.

    d. The report calls for media and communications firms to consult with IRBs prior to formal submission of recruitment materials.

3. The Office of the Inspector General Reports on recruitment call for independent lay members of an IRB to be

    a. Increased to a minimum of one third of the total membership

    b. More extensively represented

    c. Trained more rigorously in scientific methods

    d. Patient advocates

4. The issues of greatest concern for IRBs and for IRB staffs relating to recruitment campaigns are

    a. Consent (ongoing or continuing)

    b. Completeness (accuracy as well as truthfulness vs. deception)

    c. Coercion (of medium and message)

    d. All of the above

5. When a recruitment campaign is being used, the most appropriate action for an IRB is to

    a. Dictate the recruitment plan

    b. Review the full recruitment plan prior to initiation

    c. Not review the full recruitment plan

    d. Not review the full recruitment plan, only the patient screening scripts

Chapter 5-7

Advertisements for Research

1. An investigator from Central Hospital wants to post a recruitment flyer in a specialty clinic at Western Hospital. The flyer is intended to solicit volunteer subjects for the investigator's study at Central Hospital. All procedures related to the study will be conducted at Central Hospital, but there is a potential group of subjects from the specialty clinic at Western Hospital who may be eligible and/or appropriate for the study. Choose the statement that best describes the mechanism for IRB review of the protocol and recruitment flyer:

    a. The IRB at Western Hospital should be contacted to determine whether its IRB needs to review the protocol and/or recruitment flyer.

    b. IRB review of the protocol and/or recruitment flyer at Western Hospital would never be required.

    c. IRB review of the protocol and/or recruitment flyer at Western Hospital is always required.

    d. Neither Central Hospital nor Western Hospital needs to review the recruitment flyer.

2. Choose the answer that most accurately reflects the appropriate procedure for the submission of media advertisements to the IRB:

    a. Media research advertisements must be reviewed and approved by the IRB before implementation.

    b. If the protocol and consent form have been approved, it is not necessary to submit media advertisements for review.

    c. Media advertisements do not need to be submitted to the IRB prior to use but should be submitted with the annual renewal information.

    d. IRBs only need to review a brief summary of the media advertisement, and not the entire video, script, and so forth.

3. A principal investigator would like to post a clinical trial listing on the website for the Hypertension Association. Patients with hypertension frequently visit this site. The listing she would like to post is as follows:

    The following study is being conducted at Best Hospital:

    "A Multicenter Phase II Clinical Trial to Evaluate the Efficacy of HyperTDrugA for the Treatment of Hypertension in the Adult Population

    If you are interested in participating in this clinical trial, please contact Sally Smith, RN, MPH, of the Best Hospital, phone number: (123) 456–7890."

    What are the steps the principal investigator should take before posting this clinical trial listing on the Internet?

a. Because it is not a federal requirement for clinical trial listings to receive IRB approval, the principal investigator does not have to contact her IRB and the principal investigator can post the clinical trial listing on the website without contacting her IRB office.

b. Because it is a federal requirement for clinical trial listings to receive IRB approval, the principal investigator must submit the clinical trial listing to her IRB office for review and approval before posting the clinical trial listing on the website.

c. The principal investigator should contact her IRB office to determine whether IRB review and approval is required as institutional policies may indicate that listings of research studies on the Internet require IRB approval.

d. It is not appropriate for the principal investigator to post a clinical trial listing for a study that is industry-sponsored on a nonprofit website; therefore, the principal investigator will not be able to post the clinical trial listing on this website.

4. An investigator wants to have employers distribute a survey to their employees. Which is the most appropriate mechanism that should be used?

a. The supervisor personally distributes the survey to the employees and asks that they return completed surveys to the supervisor.

b. The surveys are mailed to the employees and then returned to the supervisor.

c. The surveys are mailed to the employees and then returned directly to the investigator.

d. The surveys are distributed at a staff meeting, and the employees are advised about the importance of completing the survey.

5. Potential research subjects should not feel coerced to participate in a study. Select the scenario that best illustrates this concept:

a. A clinician recommends that his patients participate in a minimal risk clinical trial for which he or she is an investigator.

b. A clinician describes a new clinical trial, for which he or she is an investigator, to his or her patients and provides them with information to take home and review.

c. A clinician leaves IRB-approved recruitment brochures for a new clinical trial in the clinic lobby. Interested individuals may contact the research coordinator at their convenience to discuss the trial.

d. A clinician asks one of his or her nurses to speak to patients about a new clinical trial for which he or she is an investigator.

Chapter 5–8

Paying Research Subjects

1. It can be argued that payment of research subjects may result in economically disadvantaged persons bearing a disproportionately large share of the risks of research. This concern is most strongly associated with which of the ethical principles described in *The Belmont Report*?

   a. Respect for persons

   b. Beneficience

   c. Nonmaleficence

   d. Justice

2. DHHS regulations (45 CFR 46) as well as guidance from OHRP

   a. Specifically prohibit payment of research subjects.

   b. Specifically recommend financial remuneration to cover reimbursement of direct costs to the subject.

   c. Require investigators to minimize the possibility of coercion or undue influence.

   d. Provide specific guidance regarding the definition of undue influence.

3. FDA regulations and guidance

   a. Endorse payment to subjects, especially in the early phases of investigational drug, biologic, or device development.

   b. Charge IRBs with the responsibility to review payment to assure that it does not represent undue influence.

   c. Consider payment to research subjects for participation in studies to be a benefit of participating.

   d. Specifically require IRBs to consider payment in their assessment of the risk–benefit relationship.

4. Which of the following is true of the reimbursement model of Dickert and Grady?

   a. It increases the risk that potential subjects withhold information to avoid being excluded from the study.

   b. It is likely to attract financially disadvantaged potential subjects.

   c. It is based on the view that research participation should be revenue neutral for participants.

   d. It is likely to accrue subjects more rapidly than other models.

5. Regarding prorating of payments to research subjects, which of the following is true?

   a. FDA regulations and guidance require prorating payments based on the duration of participation of the subject in the research.

   b. Prorating schemes may be structured to induce subjects to continue in the research study through completion.

   c. FDA only requires prorating of payment if withdrawal of the subject was involuntary (that is, based on some withdrawal criteria of the research protocol).

   d. FDA regulations specifically prohibit completion bonuses.

Chapter 5-9

Provisions for Data Monitoring

1. Choose the most accurate statement:

   a. Federal regulations require the IRB to determine that the research plan makes adequate provisions for the ongoing monitoring of study data to protect the welfare of research participants.

   b. Federal regulations require the IRB to function as a Data and Safety Monitoring Board (DSMB).

   c. Federal regulations require that the IRB compares the observed to expected rates of adverse events in each research study.

   d. Federal guidance documents, such as the 1999 National Cancer Institute (NCI) policy statement, prohibit an individual investigator from serving as the primary mechanism for data monitoring.

2. Choose the most accurate statement:

   a. According to the 1999 National Institutes of Health (NIH) policy statement, IRBs should not expect to receive information regarding DSMB deliberations until after the study is completed.

   b. Both DHHS and FDA regulations require an independent DSMB for any phase III trial.

   c. A 1999 NIH policy statement is "Once a DSMB is established, each IRB should be informed of the operating procedures with regard to data and safety monitoring (e.g., who, what, when, where, and how monitoring will take place). If the IRB is not satisfied with the monitoring procedures, it should request modifications. . . . The DSMB's summary report should provide feedback at regular and defined intervals to the IRBs."

   d. A year 2000 Office for Protection from Research Risks (OPRR) clarification letter warns that IRBs are not permitted to rely on a current statement from a DSMB regarding analysis of study-wide adverse events or interim findings but instead must review all data related to these issues at the full committee meeting.

3. Choose the most accurate statement:

   a. Federal regulations require that the IRB function as a data monitoring committee from the standpoint of comparing observed and expected rates of adverse events.

   b. The IRB should require a detailed description of stopping rules regarding the potential outcomes of the study that are likely to have a major impact on the rights or welfare of research participants.

   c. Federal guidance documents state that independent DSMBs should be required for all industry-sponsored trials.

   d. Federal policy statements make it clear that there should be no communication between data monitoring committees, such as DSMBs, and the IRB until the study is completed.

4. Which statement sets forth the best case for the IRB to require an independent DSMB for approval of research?

   a. The study involves a single site and a large number of subjects.

   b. The study involves a single site, a small number of subjects, little risk to subjects, and the investigator is not available to do data monitoring.

   c. The study is a Phase I trial.

   d. The study is a Phase III trial, involves multiple sites, a large number of subjects, and complex data analysis.

Chapter 5-10

Conflict of Interest: Researchers

1. If someone has a conflict of interest, it means that he or she has

    a. Gotten into a situation where his/her motives may be questioned

    b. Done something wrong

    c. Taken money for doing something that should have been done for free

    d. Harmed research subjects

2. Conflicts of interest are

    a. Less of a problem today than in previous decades

    b. Easy to avoid if one works in an academic setting, for a predetermined salary

    c. Inherent in many types of clinical research and may be difficult to eliminate

    d. Best controlled by disclosure to the sponsor

3. Managing conflicts of interest in research

    a. Should vary depending on the level of trust the IRB has in a given investigator

    b. Should focus on the facts and not on the IRB's perception of the conflicted individual

    c. Is easier when the investigator in question has a high level of personal integrity

    d. Should be handled differently if the conflicted person is a respected department chair or a trainee that no one knows

4. Conflicts of interest on the part of investigators should be

    a. Considered a problem only if the opportunity for personal gain is acted on

    b. Disclosed after a study is completed

    c. Disclosed only to the IRB

    d. Minimized to avoid even the perception of biased judgment

5. Which of the following best describes an investigator with a conflict of interest?

    a. It may be difficult for the investigator to recognize his or her own situation as a problem.

    b. The investigator is in the best position of anyone to recognize and manage the conflict.

    c. It is impossible for the investigator to conduct ethical research under any circumstances.

    d. The investigator must not serve on an IRB.

Chapter 5-11

Conflict of Interest: Recruitment Incentives

1. Which of the following does NOT create a potential conflict of interest?

   a. Authorship on a paper, for those investigators who enroll the most subjects

   b. A referral fee, for a general practitioner who gives his specialist colleague a list of patients eligible for a clinical trial

   c. A policy that any payments to researchers should be reviewed by the IRB

   d. An enrollment bonus paid to study coordinators, but not to the principal investigator

2. Recruitment of subjects into clinical trials is

   a. A process immune from financial incentives that might influence other aspects of the study

   b. A source of pressure for investigators and sponsors with deadlines to meet

   c. Outside of the IRB's purview

   d. Dependent on demands by subjects for payment

Chapter 5-12

Conflict of Interest: Institutional Review Boards

1. One of the most effective means for an IRB to minimize the degree that it will be subjected to institutional conflicts of interest is to

   a. Appoint university legal counsel as a member

   b. Have a chaplain or priest as a member

   c. Hold meetings that are closed to the public

   d. Appoint a diverse membership, including those from outside the institution

2. The federal regulations that govern IRB procedures

   a. Require that members with a conflict of interest not participate in the vote on that study

   b. Require that members with a conflict of interest leave the room during discussion of that study

   c. Are completely silent on the question of members who may have a conflict of interest

   d. Address only the situation in which a member serves as investigator of a research project under review

3. Which of the following best describes the IRB?

   a. It is relatively sheltered from conflict of interest issues because its main role is to provide ethical oversight.

   b. It is relatively sheltered from conflict of interest issues provided it does not receive payment for review.

   c. It should be aware of and manage factors that may influence its decisions.

   d. It can only function effectively if members have no research experience themselves.

Chapter 5–13

Administrative Tasks Before Each Institutional Review Board Meeting

1. The IRB office needs to canvass IRB members to ensure that

   a. A majority of members are present, including one member whose primary concerns are in the nonscientific area.

   b. Five members will be attending.

   c. A comfortable meeting space is reserved in proper time.

   d. The number of members is not less than the alternate members.

2. For review of a new study submission, IRB committee members need to receive

   a. An agenda listing the new protocol title and the investigator name

   b. A letter from the investigator stating his or her intention to open a study at his or her institution

   c. Study protocol, consent form, and other relevant material

   d. Consent form only

3. When an investigator submits a study for full-committee review

   a. Federal regulations require that the investigator attend the IRB meeting.

   b. Federal regulations do not allow nonmembers to attend an IRB meeting.

   c. Federal regulations require that IRB members do not discuss submissions with the investigators prior to the meeting.

   d. IRB members, including primary reviewers and the IRB office staff, may contact the researcher directly with questions before the meeting or to request further information from the researcher.

4. The IRB office staff will aid the study renewal process if the following is done BEFORE the full-committee meeting:

   a. Update the database with the new approval date for all studies to be reviewed for renewal.

   b. Notify researchers of the date that full-IRB renewal of their study is required if they wish to proceed with uninterrupted participant enrollment.

   c. Complete the study renewal form on behalf of the investigator.

   d. Provide renewal materials only to the primary reviewers of the study.

Chapter 5-14

Guidelines for Review, Discussion, and Voting

1. Choose the practice that is most likely to improve IRB function:

   a. Primary IRB reviewers have questions answered and concerns addressed before the IRB meeting.

   b. The IRB never asks a researcher to be present to discuss issues with the IRB committee.

   c. Most of the time at the full-committee meeting is spent polishing the wording of the consent document.

   d. All studies are tabled or not approved at least once to make researchers work hard for every IRB approval determination.

2. Review templates or worksheets

   a. Are not recommended because every IRB member should evaluate a study according to different criteria

   b. Should be sent to the investigator with the IRB reviewer's name on it so the investigator knows who reviewed the protocol

   c. Are likely to be useful in directing attention to the main issues that the IRB should evaluate and documenting that a substantive IRB review has taken place

   d. Should never be kept as part of the permanent IRB record because it could be used in a lawsuit

3. Choose the most accurate statement:

   a. An IRB member who is also the principal investigator of a study being reviewed by the IRB should be permitted to participate in the IRB vote on the study as long as the IRB member has no financial holdings in the sponsor of the study in question.

   b. An IRB that requires six members for a meeting quorum is conducting a meeting with seven members present. Two members have a conflict of interest that requires that they abstain from voting. The remaining IRB members may approve the study as long as it is a unanimous vote.

   c. An IRB member not allowed to vote because of a conflict of interest should leave the room for the final discussion and voting on the study in question.

   d. An IRB that requires six members for a meeting quorum is conducting a meeting with seven members present. The results of the vote on a particular study are three approve, three disapprove, and one abstain. In this situation, federal regulations require that the IRB approve the study.

Chapter 5-15

Administrative Tasks After Each Institutional Review Board Meeting

1. Minutes of the IRB meeting shall

   a. Be written as detailed as possible, describing verbatim the member's statements; the actions taken by the IRB; the IRB vote, including the number of members voting for, against, and abstaining; and the basis for requiring changes in and disapproving research.

   b. Be written in sufficient detail to show attendance at the meetings; actions taken by the IRB; the IRB vote, including the number of members voting for, against, and abstaining; the basis for requiring changes in or disapproving research; and a written summary of the discussion of controverted issues and their resolution.

   c. Be written as concisely as possible. It is not necessary to summarize the issues discussed as long as you include the resolution; the IRB vote, including the number of members voting for, against, and abstaining; and the basis for requiring changes in or disapproving research.

   d. Include only those items determined necessary by the board as long as you include the IRB vote, including who voted for, voted against, and abstained and whether the project was approved, disapproved, or required modification.

2. What statement best describes the attitude of a compliance official as it relates to documentation?

   a. If it is not documented, then it was not done.

   b. If you document everything, then there is a better chance of our finding something wrong; thus, be as concise as possible.

   c. Documentation is the most important task conducted by IRB administrators.

   d. Documentation is the root of all evil.

3. According to 45 CFR 46.115(b), records relating to research shall be retained

   a. At least 5 years after the final data has been analyzed. All records must be accessible for inspection and copying by authorized representatives of the department or agency at reasonable times and in a reasonable manner.

   b. Research records must be kept for a period determined by the sponsor of the research. All records must be accessible for inspection and copying by authorized representatives of the sponsor at reasonable times and in a reasonable manner.

   c. At least 3 years after completion of the research. All records must be accessible for inspection and copying by authorized representatives of the department or agency at reasonable times and in a reasonable manner.

   d. Research records must be kept for a period determined by the IRB and is based on the level of risk to the participants. All records must be accessible for inspection and copying by authorized representatives of the sponsor at reasonable times and in a reasonable manner.

ANSWER KEY FOR PART 5

Answer Key: Chapter 5-1

1. a
2. e
3. c
4. b

Answer Key: Chapter 5-2

1. c
2. c
3. d

Answer Key: Chapter 5-3

1. c
2. d
3. a
4. d

Answer Key: Chapter 5-4

1. c
2. b
3. c
4. d

Answer Key: Chapter 5-5

1. c
2. b
3. c
4. a
5. c
6. a

Answer Key: Chapter 5-6

1. a
2. c
3. b
4. d
5. b

Answer Key: Chapter 5-7

1. a
2. a
3. c
4. c
5. c

Answer Key: Chapter 5-8

1. d
2. c
3. b
4. c
5. a

Answer Key: Chapter 5-9

1. a
2. c
3. b
4. d

Answer Key: Chapter 5-10

1. a
2. c
3. b
4. d
5. a

Answer Key: Chapter 5-11

1. c
2. b

Answer Key: Chapter 5-12

1. d
2. a
3. c

Answer Key: Chapter 5-13

1. a
2. c
3. d
4. b

Answer Key: Chapter 5-14

1. a
2. c
3. c

Answer Key: Chapter 5-15

1. b
2. a
3. c

Part 6

Informed Consent

Chapter 6-1

The Institutional Review Board's Role in Editing the Consent Document

1. Choose the statement that most accurately reflects the author's opinion about the role of the institutional review board (IRB) in editing the consent document:

   a. It is appropriate for IRBs to edit the consent document.

   b. The IRB should not attempt to edit the consent document.

   c. Federal regulations direct the IRB to send inadequate consent documents back to the investigator with a directive to "rewrite the consent document in lay language."

   d. An investigator who submits a sloppy consent document should be penalized by having approval of the study delayed for at least 2 months.

2. With which of the following statements would the author be likely to agree?

   a. Designating a single IRB member to act as a primary "consent editor" might be an efficient way for IRBs to organize consent reviews.

   b. The consent process is more important than the consent document.

   c. Because subjects get an opportunity to ask questions, it is not important that the consent document be easily understandable.

   d. Investigators and sponsors just ignore consent templates and drafting instructions and samples so that it is a waste of time for IRBs to prepare and post them on their websites.

3. Which of the following is NOT suggested in the author's chapter?

   a. In its response to the investigator, the IRB should distinguish between "suggested" language changes and "required" language changes.

   b. The IRB should not wait until it reviews the consent document before telling investigators about standard language it requires for such situations as pregnancy testing, videotaping, or placebos. Instead, any standard, required language should be included in the IRB's submission instructions.

   c. The IRB should be willing to entertain alternative language from the investigator that communicates the necessary information clearly. The IRB should only insist that investigators use the IRB's preferred wording if alternate phrasings would be truly unacceptable.

   d. IRBs should not bother preparing template consents or standard language for common procedures since the IRB always has to ask for lots of changes to the consent document anyway.

Chapter 6-2

The Consent Document

1. The consent document

    a. Should describe every conceivable event and risk that a subject could possibly encounter from research participation

    b. Should be long so that the subject will understand everything they need to know

    c. Should be limited to the information that a reasonable person would want to know to decide about research participation

    d. Should downplay risks, as this may discourage research participation

2. The IRB's role in reviewing consent is best described as

    a. IRB reviewers should not revise the consent document as needed before the meeting. It is better to make the investigator figure out what the IRB needs to approve the study at a future meeting.

    b. Polishing the wording of the consent document is a productive and important use of full-committee meeting time.

    c. The IRB should not use auto text language in the consent document that has been approved previously by the IRB for use in specific situations.

    d. The IRB should use a system whereby an experienced reviewer revises the consent document as needed before the full-committee meeting.

3. After the investigator has made the changes to the consent document recommended by the IRB, the following steps should be taken:

    a. The investigator should send a notice to the IRB that the consent form has been changed. The IRB should stamp the originally submitted consent form "approved" with an expiration date.

    b. The investigator should resubmit the written, revised consent form for final approval.

    c. The investigator should resubmit the written, revised consent form to the IRB. If the IRB determines that it meets all requirements, the form should be stamped "approved" on every page.

Chapter 6-3

Exculpatory Language in Informed Consent Documents

1. The prohibition on "exculpatory language" in informed consent

    a. Does not appear in the Federal Policy (Common Rule) for the Protection of Human Subjects

    b. Applies only to Food and Drug Administration (FDA)–regulated research

    c. Applies to Department of Health and Human Services (DHHS)–supported research, but not to DHHS-conducted research

    d. Applies to all research governed by the Common Rule, DHHS regulations, or FDA regulations

2. According to DHHS, "exculpatory language"

    a. Includes only language that would release the institution/investigator from liability for wrongful acts

    b. Describes the reimbursement that the investigator can receive from the study sponsor

    c. Includes any language through which the subject is made to waive, or appear to waive, any of the subject's legal rights

    d. Describes the investigator's right to penalize the subject for poor compliance with the protocol

3. DHHS regulations permit informed consent language that

    a. Says that the institution has no policy or plan to pay for injuries that the subject receives as a result of participating

    b. Holds the institution/investigator "harmless"

    c. Holds the sponsor "harmless"

    d. Describes the subject's voluntary agreement not to sue the investigator/institution

4. In a practical sense, exculpatory statements tend to be

    a. More favorable to the subject than to the investigator/institution

    b. Statements in which a subject is asked to agree to or accept something

    c. Valid only in states that have a formal "Subjects' Bill of Rights"

    d. Statements that set forth simple facts

Chapter 6-4

Requiring a Witness Signature on the Consent Form

1. The signature of a witness on the standard (long form) informed consent document

    a. Is required by federal regulations for research participation

    b. Indicates that the witness was present during the entire consent conference

    c. Is not required by federal regulations when the (standard long form) consent document is signed by the subject or the subject's legally authorized representative

    d. Is required by federal regulations when consent is obtained from a subject's legally authorized representative

2. Under federal regulations, the signature of a witness on a "short form" informed consent document

    a. Indicates that the witness observed the oral presentation of informed consent information

    b. Is the only signature needed when consent information is presented orally

    c. Is valid only if the witness is a member of the research team

    d. Indicates that the subject understood what was presented orally

3. When state laws provide protections for subjects that go beyond those required under federal regulations

    a. The federal requirements automatically override the state requirements.

    b. The state requirements must be observed.

    c. FDA or OHRP can waive the state requirements after publishing an announcement in the *Federal Register.*

    d. Institutional policy determines which protections to use.

4. When a witness signature is used on the standard (long form) informed consent document

    a. The signature of the investigator is also required.

    b. The subject need not be given a copy of the document.

    c. The witness should sign before the subject signs.

    d. Best practice suggests that it should include a description of what the signature means.

5. The date of the signature of the subject or the subject's legally authorized representative on the consent document

    a. Is optional

    b. Is required under FDA regulations

    c. Is required under DHHS regulations

    d. Both (b) and (c)

Chapter 6-5

Deception of Research Subjects

1. The main argument against the use of research involving deception of research subjects is that

   a. Deception of research subjects makes it impossible to generate meaningful research results.

   b. Deception is not needed to study human behavior.

   c. Deception in research may be unethical, potentially harmful to research participants, harmful to the researcher's profession, and ultimately harmful to society.

   d. Role playing by research subjects is an effective alternative to deception.

2. Choose the most accurate statement:

   a. Deception is never harmful when the subject is debriefed after the study.

   b. An IRB should never consider the trade-off between the risk of deceiving an individual subject and the potential benefit of the research to other members of society.

   c. It is impossible to study certain aspects of human behavior without deception of research subjects.

   d. Federal regulations state that deception of subjects is acceptable in social science research but not in biomedical research.

3. According to the American Psychological Association, the three requirements for deception in research are

   a. Estimation of a favorable cost/benefit profile of the research.

   Deception is required to answer the research question.

   Fully explain the nature of the deception at the conclusion of the study or present a compelling justification for withholding such information.

   b. The principal investigator has experience with research involving deception.

   Deception is required to answer the research question.

   Fewer subjects are required with, than without, deceptive techniques.

   c. It will be difficult to enroll subjects without deception.

   Fully explain the nature of the deception at the conclusion of the study.

   Deception is required to answer the research question.

   d. Estimation of a favorable cost/benefit profile of the research.

   Deception is required to answer the research question.

   It will be difficult to enroll subjects without deception.

4. Choose the most accurate statement:

   a. It is often acceptable to deceive subjects about the confidentiality of research information.

   b. Debriefing subjects at the conclusion of the study usually causes more harm than good.

   c. Deception is often used when there is the potential for physical harm.

   d. A requirement in the code of the American Psychological Association that may generate disagreement between the IRB and the investigator is the requirement that researchers cannot deceive prospective participants regarding "research that is reasonably expected to cause physical pain or severe emotional distress."

Chapter 6-6

Research Without Consent or Documentation Thereof

1. What situation is most likely to qualify for waiver of informed consent?

   a. Research to evaluate prospectively a new material for repairing dental cavities

   b. Research that tests donated blood for evidence of illegal drug use

   c. Research that involves retrospective review of data from the medical record to evaluate outcome following elective pregnancy termination (abortion)

   d. Research that involves retrospective review of data from the medical record to evaluate outcome following hip replacement surgery

2. Which situation is most likely to qualify for waiver of documentation of informed consent because documentation places the subject at risk of harm?

   a. Face-to-face interview of rape victims

   b. Face-to-face interview of heart transplant recipients

   c. Face-to-face interview of mothers of twins to evaluate the desire to have more children

   d. Face-to-face interview of cancer survivors

3. The criteria for waiving the requirement for documentation of informed consent according to DHHS regulations at 45 CFR 46.117(c) are

   a. A signed consent document would put the subject at risk of harm if there was a breach in confidentiality, AND the research is minimal risk and does not involve procedures for which signed consent is normally required.

   b. A signed consent document would put the subject at risk of harm if there was a breach in confidentiality, OR the research is minimal risk and does not involve procedures for which signed consent is normally required.

   c. A signed consent document would put the subject at risk of harm if there was a breach in confidentiality, AND it is impracticable for the investigator to get documentation of informed consent.

   d. It is impracticable for the investigator to get documentation of informed consent, OR the research is minimal risk and does not involve procedures for which signed consent is normally required.

4. Choose the statement that most accurately completes the following statement:
   When the IRB approves a waiver of informed consent or a waiver of documentation of consent

   a. There are no specific documentation requirements.

   b. The IRB meeting minutes must document the determination to grant the waiver.

   c. The IRB meeting minutes, or in the case of expedited review, the expedited reviewer, must document the specific findings required by the regulations, which demonstrate that a waiver is justified.

   d. The subjects must be notified.

Chapter 6-7

Selecting a Surrogate to Consent to Medical Research

1. Choose the answer that most accurately applies to IRB approval of research in which the participant is not competent to give informed consent:

   a. Federal regulations state that informed consent for research must be obtained from a "next-of-kin" if the subjects are not competent to give informed consent themselves.

   b. DHHS regulations at 45 CFR 46.111(a)(4) require informed consent from each prospective subject or the subject's legally authorized representative, but "legally authorized" in the context of medical research is often not defined.

   c. Most states have laws explaining that any close relative is legally authorized to give informed consent for an incompetent subject to participate in research.

   d. Federal Regulations require informed consent from a court-appointed guardian to involve an incompetent subject in medical research.

2. Choose the most accurate statement:

   a. In all states, a "next-of-kin" is legally authorized to give consent for an incompetent person to participate in research.

   b. In all states, the "caregiver" of a person with severe dementia is legally authorized to give consent for the demented person to participate in research.

   c. Some states have family consent laws that specify a hierarchy of surrogate decision makers for healthcare decisions.

   d. In all states, a court-appointed guardian of a demented person is legally authorized to give consent for the demented person to participate in research.

Chapter 6-8

Research-Related Injuries

1. Under the Code of Federal Regulations, when an individual sustains a research-related injury, research institutions are required to

    a. Provide free medical care to injured research subjects

    b. Have explained before participation whether medical treatments are available

    c. Provide compensation to the injured research participant

    d. Notify the institution's legal counsel for advice on how to proceed

2. IRB members and administrators should keep certain issues in mind before deliberating about subject protection requirements in case of research-related injury:

    a. An IRB can only suggest that a principal investigator consider whether to provide free medical care in case of injury.

    b. First and foremost, IRBs have to protect themselves from liability for research-related injury.

    c. IRBs have the legal authority to mandate provision of free medical care when the risk justifies it.

    d. IRBs should depend on the study sponsor for any risk/benefit analysis it might need.

3. The fourth provision of the Nuremberg Code addresses the issue of compensation for research-related injuries. It reads as follows:

    a. The degree of risk to be taken should never exceed that determined by the humanitarian importance of the problem to be solved by the experiment.

    b. No experiment should be conducted where there is an a priori reason to believe that death or disabling injury will occur, except, perhaps, in those experiments where the experimental physicians also serve as subjects.

    c. The voluntary consent of the human subject is absolutely essential.

    d. The experiment should be so conducted as to avoid all unnecessary physical and mental suffering and injury.

4. Provision of medical care for research-related injury is an issue in this country because the United States

    a. Has the highest proportion of research-related injury in the world

    b. Has a severe health care professional shortage

    c. Does not have adequate governmental health insurance oversight

    d. Does not have a national health insurance program

5. Concern over compensation for research-related injury has recently become a prominent concern for the international research protections community after being overshadowed by which issue for the last decade?

   a. Imbalance of power

   b. Comparable standard of care

   c. Equitable distribution of research outcomes

   d. Complexity of informed consent

6. The general argument made at the international level for the need for research-related injury compensation centers around the precept of

   a. Reasonable availability

   b. Informed consent

   c. Fair benefits

   d. Capacity building

Chapter 6-9

Informing Subjects about Research Results

1. What do federal regulations (45 CFR 46) require about informing research subjects about research findings?

   a. If the information may directly benefit the subject, subjects must be informed.

   b. Because research information is speculative and the implications of the information for the individual subject are unclear, subjects must not be informed.

   c. If research findings will affect the subject's decision to continue participation in the study, subjects must be informed.

   d. Research subjects should always have a choice whether to be informed.

2. Subjects in a study will have their urine analyzed for sugar to determine the incidence of diabetes in a large population. Sugar in the urine accurately predicts people with diabetes. Investigators will have access to the identity of each subject linked to the urinalysis result. Should the investigators inform subjects about their own research results?

   a. All subjects should be informed.

   b. No subjects should be informed.

   c. Subjects should choose whether they want to be informed.

   d. Results should be given to the subject's physician but not to the subject.

3. Subjects in a study will have blood drawn to test for a particular gene. The presence of the gene may predict the development of pancreatic cancer, but this is very preliminary and speculative. Investigators will have access to the identity of each subject linked to the DNA result. Should the investigators inform subjects about their own research results?

   a. All subjects should be informed.

   b. No subjects should be informed.

   c. Subjects should choose whether they want to be informed.

   d. Results should be given to the subject's physician but not to the subject.

Chapter 6-10

Explaining the Costs of Research Participation

1. The author recommends that the informed consent document

    a. State that the subject's insurance company will pay for research-related expenses.

    b. State that the sponsor will pay for research-related expenses.

    c. State specifically which expenses will be charged to the insurance company, which expenses will be charged to the sponsor, and which expenses the subject may be at risk to pay.

    d. Distinguish which services are considered part of the standard of care and which are conducted to advance research objectives.

Chapter 6-11

Improving Informed Consent

1. The author suggests that to evaluate quality of informed consent one must consider three areas. Which area should not be considered?

   a. Structure

   b. Length

   c. Outcome

   d. Process

2. Process refers to

   a. Tangible elements required for a good informed consent

   b. Actual results of a high-quality informed consent

   c. Actions necessary to obtain high-quality consent

   d. Revising an informed consent document

3. In the final analysis, which element is most important in improving the quality of informed consent?

   a. Structure

   b. Process

   c. Outcome

   d. Benchmarking

4. Comprehension in the informed consent process requires the ability to

   a. Memorize an informed consent document

   b. Interpret the knowledge imparted

   c. Sign the consent document

   d. Understand the risks and benefits section of the consent only

5. The author refers to benchmarking as a method to assist in improving the informed consent process. An example of benchmarking would be

   a. Measuring the outcome of the consent process against other institutions

   b. Speaking with research subjects to see how well they understood the consent form

   c. Asking investigators to do a better job of explaining the research

   d. Offering a seminar to investigators on the informed consent process

6. The author refers to four steps to improve the quality of the informed consent process. They are listed here in random order. Which step would need to be taken first?

   a. Implement an intervention to improve informed consent.

   b. Monitor the effectiveness of an intervention to improve informed consent.

   c. Act on results of measurements that evaluate informed consent.

   d. Establish a baseline measurement for quality of informed consent.

Chapter 6-12

Informed Consent Evaluation Feedback Tool

1. Choose the most accurate statement:

    a. The authors of this chapter recommend that the research subject sign the Informed Consent Evaluation Feedback Tool (ICE FT) to document compliance with federal regulations.

    b. It is well documented that most research participants view the consent document as their primary source of information about the study.

    c. Using a tool like the ICE FT, either before or after the initial discussion, may improve the quality of informed consent.

    d. It is best to test the quality of informed consent a few weeks after research participation has started.

ANSWER KEY FOR PART 6

Answer Key: Chapter 6-1

1. a
2. a
3. d

Answer Key: Chapter 6-2

1. c
2. d
3. c

Answer Key: Chapter 6-3

1. d
2. c
3. a
4. b

Answer Key: Chapter 6-4

1. c
2. a
3. b
4. d
5. b

Answer Key: Chapter 6-5

1. c
2. c
3. a
4. d

Answer Key: Chapter 6-6

1. d
2. a
3. b
4. c

Answer Key: Chapter 6-7

1. b
2. c

Answer Key: Chapter 6-8

1. b
2. c
3. d
4. d
5. b
6. c

Answer Key: Chapter 6-9

1. c
2. a
3. b

Answer Key: Chapter 6-10

1. c

Answer Key: Chapter 6-11

1. b
2. c
3. c
4. b
5. a
6. d

Answer Key: Chapter 6-12

1. c

Part 7

Continuing Review

Chapter 7-1

Revisions to Approved Study

1. Which of the following protocol revisions would most likely qualify for expedited institutional review board (IRB) review?

    a. Adding the risk of cardiac abnormalities to the consent form

    b. Expanding the eligibility criteria to include children in addition to adults

    c. Adding a new investigational drug to the research intervention

    d. Deleting two questions from a 10-page survey instrument

2. Revised consent forms may be used as soon as

    a. The sponsor says it is okay to use the revised consent form

    b. The IRB staff screens the incoming consent document for accuracy

    c. The principal investigator identifies a patient that qualifies for the study

    d. The IRB has provided approval of the revised consent document

3. Which IRB review mechanism is required for changes to the protocol involving major risks?

    a. Approval by the IRB chair only

    b. Approval by the IRB chair and/or a qualified member of the IRB

    c. Approval by the sponsor and a letter of support addressed to the IRB

    d. Full IRB review at a convened meeting

4. A protocol revision approved by the IRB is effective for what period of time?

    a. 365 days beyond the date of approval

    b. Eleven months beyond the date of approval

    c. The length of time specified by the investigator in the initial request for IRB review of the protocol revision

    d. Until the expiration date of the most recent continuation review for the protocol

Chapter 7-2

Protocol Renewal

1. Choose the most accurate statement:

   a. Only the primary reviewer should receive a copy of the protocol and current consent document at the time of continuation review. It is not necessary to burden other IRB members with this information.

   b. The criteria for IRB approval at the time of continuation review are the same as they were at initial review.

   c. Federal regulations require continuation review on each protocol at least every 2 years.

   d. The criteria for IRB approval at the time of continuation review are less demanding than those used at the time of initial review.

2. Choose the answer that most accurately describes a situation in which a protocol that initially required full-committee IRB review may undergo continuation review with an expedited process:

   a. The protocol is revised so that future interventions are less risky than the interventions that were previously approved by the full IRB committee.

   b. The protocol is closed to new enrollment, and 95% of the subjects have completed research interventions without ill effects.

   c. Analysis of previously enrolled subjects suggests that the risk of research participation is no more than minimal.

   d. Research is permanently closed to enrollment, all subjects have completed research-related interventions, and research remains active only for long-term follow-up.

3. IRB protocol renewal review is required per regulation at least

   a. Twice every 365 days

   b. Three times every 365 days

   c. Once every 365 days

   d. Quarterly every 365 days

4. If a protocol was initially reviewed and approved using an expedited review procedure, which of the following best describes the protocol renewal requirements?

   a. Renewal and review by the IRB is not required.

   b. Renewal and review by the IRB is required at a convened meeting.

   c. Renewal and review can be managed by IRB staff.

   d. Renewal and review by the IRB may continue under the expedited review process provided there were no changes to the protocol.

5. Which of the following IRB actions would be required when an investigator fails to meet IRB protocol renewal requirements?

   a. Suspend study

   b. Send a second notice to the investigator

   c. Provide a study extension authorized by the chair

   d. Re-review the most recent IRB-approved study documents

Chapter 7-3

Institutional Review Board Review of Adverse Events

1. Department of Health and Human Services (DHHS) and Food and Drug Administration (FDA) regulations for the protection of human subjects require adverse events be reported to the IRB

   a. Immediately

   b. Promptly

   c. Within 72 hours

   d. Within 1 week

2. The responsibility for interim data safety analysis in a multicenter clinical trial should rest with

   a. The FDA

   b. A Data and Safety Monitoring Board (DSMB)

   c. The Office for Human Research Protections (OHRP)

   d. The lead investigator's IRB

3. DHHS and corollary FDA regulations for research oversight require

   a. All clinical trials to establish a DSMB

   b. The IRB to conduct continuing review of research not less than once per year

   c. Sponsors of multisite clinical trials to report all adverse events directly to each IRB

   d. Prompt reporting of unanticipated risks to subjects, but not risks to "others"

4. Under the federal regulations, an unanticipated risk to which a subject is exposed is

   a. A reportable event, if there is any actual harm

   b. A reportable event, only if there is serious harm

   c. A reportable event, and actual harm is not required

   d. Not a reportable event

Chapter 7-4

Data and Safety Monitoring

1. In this chapter, the author presents five features of a research study that suggest the need for a DSMB. Choose the answer that most accurately describes three of these features:

   a. The principal investigator will benefit in some way if the study yields a positive result.

      The study population is large.

      There are high expected co-morbidity rates in the study population.

   b. The study population is large.

      There are high expected co-morbidity rates in the study population.

      There are multiple study sites.

   c. There are multiple study sites.

      It is an industry-sponsored trial.

      There are high chance of early termination.

   d. There are high expected co-morbidity rates in the study population.

      The research involves an investigational drug or device.

      There are highly toxic therapy or dangerous procedures.

2. Which statement provides the most accurate explanation of why the DSMB is in the better position to monitor the safety of subjects than IRBs?

   a. DSMBs may unblind the treatment assignments of the study subjects without compromising the objectivity of the investigator. This allows the DSMB to more easily detect excess morbidity and mortality or a clear outcome that reduces risk to subjects.

   b. Members of DSMBs are more apt to have the appropriate expertise to monitor safety.

   c. DSMBs have greater flexibility to review data at more frequent intervals.

   d. DSMBs use a more rigorous approach to monitoring safety than IRBs.

Chapter 7-5

Noncompliance, Complaints, Deviations, Eligibility Exceptions

1. What is the best way for an IRB to establish a policy on noncompliance with federal research regulations?

    a. Write a policy when you have your first reported incidence of noncompliance/complaint.

    b. Assign a committee to write the noncompliance/complaint policy.

    c. Write clear, concise procedures describing your institution's policy on noncompliance.

    d. Write general policies, because your institution needs to have some latitude in this area.

2. Who should be involved in writing the noncompliance/complaint policy?

    a. The chancellor or president of your institution

    b. The Council of Deans or CEO of your institution

    c. The IRB administrator in conjunction with the full IRB

    d. There is no one right method.

3. What should not be contained in a noncompliance/complaint policy?

    a. An outline of the procedures that the IRB will follow

    b. Guidelines for notifying Office for Human Research Protections (OHRP)

    c. The nature of the complaints that will be covered

    d. Information on types of publications that will be covered

4. What should be the first step of the noncompliance/complaint procedure?

    a. Determine whether immediate suspension of IRB approval of the study is required.

    b. Assess the whistle-blower's credibility.

    c. Set up a meeting with the sponsor.

    d. Get a list of all the investigator's publications.

5. Who needs to be notified if a study is suspended?

    a. The investigator

    b. The investigator, institutional officials, the FDA, and the OHRP, if appropriate

    c. The investigator and the department chair

    d. The chancellor/president or CEO of the institution

Chapter 7-6

Institutional Review Board Closure of Study Files

1. Which federal agency has issued guidance that requires an investigator to report the closure of a study to the IRB?

   a. FDA

   b. OHRP

   c. None

   d. Office of Civil Rights

2. According to the author, most IRBs use the following approach to study closure:

   a. Administrative closure

   b. Closure after full board review

   c. Closure by expedited review

   d. Closure by the concurrence of the chairman and vice chairman

3. Which of the following federal agencies has a specific regulation requiring the IRB to close a study after all subjects have completed the research?

   a. FDA

   b. None

   c. OHRP

   d. Office of Civil Rights

ANSWER KEY FOR PART 7

Answer Key: Chapter 7-1

1. d
2. d
3. d
4. d

Answer Key: Chapter 7-2

1. b
2. d
3. c
4. d
5. a

Answer Key: Chapter 7-3

1. b
2. b
3. b
4. c

Answer Key: Chapter 7-4

1. b
2. a

Answer Key: Chapter 7-5

1. c
2. d
3. d
4. a
5. b

Answer Key: Chapter 7-6

1. a
2. a
3. b

Part 8

Administrative and Regulatory Issues

Chapter 8-1

Health Insurance Portability and Accountability Act (HIPAA) and Research

1. An individual can give permission to use or disclose his or her protected health information through

   a. An informed consent

   b. A consent for treatment

   c. An authorization

   d. A waiver of consent

2. Under the Common Rule and Food and Drug Administration (FDA) research regulations, an institutional review board (IRB) must

   a. Review authorizations

   b. Review authorizations, only if combined with a consent for research

   c. Keep authorizations and consents separate

   d. Keep authorizations and consents together

3. In a limited data set with data use agreement, the following are allowed identifiers:

   a. Dates

   b. Names

   c. ZIP codes

   d. Both a and c

Chapter 8-2

Office for Human Research Protections Federalwide Assurance

1. An institution engaged in human subject research requires a federalwide assurance for

    a. Federally funded research

    b. Privately sponsored research

    c. FDA-regulated research

    d. An unfunded graduate student research project

2. A federalwide assurance requires the designation of a registered IRB that is

    a. In-house

    b. From another institution

    c. Independent of the institution

    d. Either in-house, from another institution, or from an independent IRB

3. Which of the following best describes the Human Protection Administrator?

    a. A high institutional official with legal authority to represent the institution

    b. A person responsible for designing investigator-training programs in human subject research protection

    c. An IRB staff member

    d. An employee or agent of the institution who exercises day-to-day operational responsibility for the program for protecting human subjects

4. A federalwide assurance includes reference to

    a. Ethical principles for domestic sites only

    b. Compliance standards for international sites only

    c. The institutional official's policy and procedures manual

    d. Ethical principles and compliance standards for either domestic institutions or international institutions

Chapter 8-3

International Conference on Harmonisation

1. Which one of the following statements best describes the "legal status" of the International Conference on Harmonisation (ICH) in the United States?

   a. The ICH has been adopted as regulation by the FDA, and compliance is mandatory for all studies under FDA jurisdiction.

   b. The ICH was enacted by the United States Congress and is a binding congressional statute in the United States Code.

   c. The ICH has been adopted as guidance by the FDA, and compliance in the United States is voluntary.

   d. The FDA has not accepted ICH, and it is not appropriate to follow ICH in the United States.

2. Which of the following statements best describes the relationship of the FDA and ICH statements on vulnerability?

   a. The ICH examples of vulnerable subjects are not the same as the FDA examples, and therefore, the ICH examples should be disregarded.

   b. Both provide incomplete lists of examples of vulnerable subjects, but both provide a useful starting point for IRBs when considering additional safeguards.

   c. The ICH definition of vulnerability applies to third-world international research only and needs to be considered in that context alone.

   d. The FDA definition and examples are relevant only to studies conducted in the United States.

3. Choose the most accurate statement regarding the ICH requirements for notification to subjects about access to medical records:

   a. ICH does not discuss this matter.

   b. ICH requires that subjects agree to have their medical records accessed by Interpol.

   c. ICH requires that subjects be notified that their research records are strictly confidential.

   d. ICH requires that subjects authorize regulatory authorities to review their research and their medical records.

4. Which of the following requirements regarding informed consent is required *only* by ICH and *not* by the FDA or Department of Health and Human Services (DHHS) regulations? The consent form must be signed and dated by

   a. The subject

   b. The person conducting the consent discussion

   c. The investigator

   d. The subject's closest living relative

5. Which of the following statements regarding the assent of incompetent subjects is most accurate?

   a. FDA and DHHS regulations do not require that incompetent adults assent to research, but ICH does require that incompetent adults assent to research when possible.

   b. ICH and the FDA and DHHS regulations all require that incompetent adults assent to research when possible.

   c. The FDA regulations and ICH require that incompetent adults assent to research when possible, but the DHHS regulations do not.

   d. The DHHS regulations and ICH require that incompetent adults assent to research when possible, but the FDA regulations do not.

6. Which of the following statements regarding "subject's responsibilities" is most accurate?

   a. The FDA and DHHS regulations and ICH all require statements about subjects' responsibilities, even though this requirement has the unintended consequence of making consent look like a contract.

   b. The FDA regulations and ICH require specific statements about subjects' responsibilities, but the DHHS regulations do not.

   c. The DHHS regulations and ICH require specific statements about subjects' responsibilities, but the FDA regulations do not.

   d. The FDA and DHHS regulations do not require any statements about subjects' responsibilities, but ICH does.

7. Which of the answers best describes the ICH requirements for the consent process when a subject or a legally acceptable representative is unable to read?

   a. The consent form should be read to the subject or the legally acceptable representative, and they may then sign and date the consent form.

   b. The consent form should be read to the subject or the legally acceptable representative, and a witness should also sign the consent form.

   c. The consent form should be read to the subject or the legally acceptable representative, and an impartial witness should be present during the entire informed consent discussion. After the written informed consent form is read and explained to the subject or the legally authorized representative, the impartial witness should sign and personally date the consent form.

   d. The consent form should be read to the subject or the legally acceptable representative, and an impartial witness (who is a family member of the subject or the legally acceptable representative) should be present during the entire informed consent discussion. After the written informed consent form is read and explained to the subject or the legally authorized representative, the impartial witness should sign and personally date the consent form.

Chapter 8-4

Gene Therapy Oversight

1. Which of the following is not recommended for review of human gene transfer experiments?

   a. Research protocol

   b. Standard operating procedures

   c. Informed consent document

   d. Investigator's brochure

2. Well-written standard operating procedures for the review of human gene tansfer experiments:

   a. Provide information on the receipt, storage, and handling of experimental agents

   b. Serve as a training guide for IRB staff

   c. Provide information for the BSO on the institutions' environmental health and safety program

   d. Provide background information on the study sponsor

3. Where is the Institutional Biosafety Committee (IBC) located?

   a. Regional offices throughout the United States

   b. Washington, D.C.

   c. At each institution

   d. Within the FDA

4. Which approval cannot be granted until RAC review is complete?

   a. FDA

   b. IRB

   c. IBC

   d. All of the above

5. What is the role of the IBC in the review of gene transfer protocols?

   a. Ensure compliance with National Institutes of Health guidelines

   b. Assess the safety of recombinant DNA research

   c. Identify any potential risk to the public health or the environment

   d. All of the above

Chapter 8-5

Understanding the Food and Drug Administration's Investigational New Drug Process

1. An investigational new drug application (IND) is always required when

   a. Newly developed drugs are tested in animals only, with no intention of involving human subjects

   b. An unlicensed agent is used in a single patient

   c. Comparing two licensed drugs in a nonsponsored research trial in which the results of the trial are intended for publication and the results are unlikely to yield a new market indication for the drugs being compared

   d. A sponsor wishes to test a new drug for safety and efficacy and, ultimately, market approval

2. If it is difficult for an investigator to determine whether an IND is required, the best resource and consultation would be with

   a. Institutional counsel

   b. The IRB chair

   c. The sponsor

   d. The FDA directly

3. Which of the following best describes the purpose of an IND?

   a. An IND provides a reliable means to assist manufacturers in reaching the potential market for a new research and development (R&D) initiative.

   b. It discourages off-label use of licensed products.

   c. An IND informs the public that prior animal studies were completed before involvement in human beings.

   d. It ensures the rights and welfare of study subjects and the quality and integrity of data on which licensing applications are based.

4. What is the most common situation in which the requirement for IRB review of an IND may be waived?

   a. When a "clinical hold" is placed on a trial

   b. If a study involves a "treatment IND"

   c. If a study involves a special waiver of consent for treatment studies conducted in an emergency setting

   d. When a treating physician wishes to use an experimental drug in a single patient for a life-threatening situation where, at a minimum, there is no standard therapy that will work and time does not permit the convening of an IRB to review the IND before its administration.

Chapter 8-6

Differences Between Department of Health and Human Services and Food and Drug Administration Regulations

1. Choose the most accurate statement:

   a. Both DHHS and FDA regulations require IRB approval to use an investigational drug in an emergency medical situation.

   b. DHHS and FDA regulations differ in the requirements for reporting adverse events.

   c. Because the FDA is part of the DHHS, an IRB that is in compliance with DHHS regulations at 45 CFR 46 is in compliance with all relevant federal regulations.

   d. DHHS regulations at 45 CFR 56 require an explicit statement in the consent document that federal authorities have the right to inspect research records.

2. This chapter discusses three areas where there are differences between DHHS regulations at 45 CFR 46 and FDA regulations at 21 CFR 50 and 56. Choose the answer that most accurately summarizes the three areas where the regulations are not identical:

   a. Criteria for exempting research from IRB review

   Criteria for IRB approval of a placebo-controlled trial

   Requirement for reporting adverse events

   b. Use of an investigational drug in an emergency medical situation

   Requirement for reporting adverse events

   Definition of a human subject

   c. Use of an investigational drug in an emergency medical situation

   Requirements for reporting adverse events

   Explaining access to study records in the consent document

   d. Requirements for reporting adverse events

   Explaining access to study records in the consent document

   Criteria for waiving the requirement for documentation of informed consent

Chapter 8-7

Veterans Administration Research Guidelines

1. A Veterans Administration (VA) facility may not use which of the following:

   a. An internal IRB

   b. An independent IRB

   c. An IRB at the affiliated not-for-profit

   d. An IRB at an affiliated university

2. Before research can be conducted at a VA facility, it must have approval of

   a. Any IRB

   b. The designated IRB for the facility at which the research will be conducted

   c. The designated IRB and the R&D committee for the facility at which the research will be conducted

   d. The R&D committee for the facility at which the research will be conducted

3. At the VA, research medication is stored

   a. As described in the protocol

   b. In the designated pharmacy

   c. At the university affiliate

   d. At the discretion of the investigator

4. Verification of credentials and annual education is required of which VA personnel?

   a. All persons working at the VA

   b. All persons engaged in research at the VA except those handling tissue or data

   c. All persons engaged in research at the VA including members of oversight committees

   d. Only research staff paid by the VA

5. VA subjects may not be paid to participate in research unless

   a. The research will directly enhance the treatment or diagnosis of the participant.

   b. There is no other way to get people to enroll.

   c. Participants in collaborating non-VA or affiliated sites are being paid.

   d. The sponsor has provided funds for payment to subjects.

6. Notwithstanding the requirements of other agencies, the VA requires the facility to maintain research records for how many years?

   a. Two years after completion of the research

   b. Three years

   c. Five years after completion of the research

   d. Three years after the drug is approved

7. At a VA facility, for-cause suspension of drug research by the IRB requires reporting to which agencies?

   a. Researchers only

   b. Office of Research Oversight (ORO), Office for Human Research Protections (OHRP), and FDA

   c. OHRP and FDA

   d. FDA only

8. VA researchers must obtain approvals from which of the following before conducting research involving children:

   a. IRB only

   b. IRB, R&D, and the Chief R&D Officer (CRADO) of the Office of Research and Development (ORD)

   c. R&D only

   d. IRB and R&D

Chapter 8-8

State Law

1. Which law determines the age of consent for participation in research?

   a. Federal law

   b. State law

   c. HIPAA

   d. FDA and OHRP regulations

2. To obtain legally valid informed consent for an incapacitated adult subject, a site should

   a. Ask a relative or spouse of the subject to sign the consent form

   b. Obtain legal advice to find out who is legally authorized to give consent in that state

   c. Refrain from enrolling any subject who has not signed a durable power of attorney for health care

   d. Have the subject sign an assent and have a relative or spouse sign the consent form

3. Which of the following are potential sources of information about state laws affecting research?

   a. 1, 3, and 4

   b. 2, 3, and 4

   c. 1, 2, and 4

   d. 3 and 4

      1. The legal department of the sponsor or contract research organization (CRO)

      2. The state department of health

      3. The OHRP

      4. Health care law attorneys

4. Which of the following must be reviewed in order to determine the privacy laws that apply to a research site:

   a. HIPAA laws and FDA regulations

   b. HIPAA laws

   c. HIPAA laws and state laws

   d. FDA regulations

Chapter 8-9

Institutional Review Board Member Liability

1. Two methods that IRBs can use to minimize financial exposure are

    a. Making certain they have adequate insurance and obtaining written indemnification from sponsors and CROs

    b. Making certain they have adequate insurance and belonging to a trade association

    c. Conducting training sessions for all members and having a paralegal as a board member

    d. Conducting training sessions for all members and having frequent internal audits

2. To indemnify means to

    a. Assume responsibility for defending all claims and paying all costs connected with reviewing studies

    b. Sign a confidentiality agreement

    c. Participate in an FDA audit

    d. Purchase malpractice insurance

3. What type of legal claim is a subject most likely to make against IRB members?

    a. Strict liability

    b. Intentional misconduct

    c. Violation of the right to be treated with dignity

    d. Negligence

4. In some states, courts have determined that the informed consent document is

    a. The law of the research study

    b. A legal contract

    c. An insurance policy

    d. A standard for imposing criminal penalties

Chapter 8-10

Certificates of Confidentiality

1. The purpose of a Certificate of Confidentiality is to

   a. Protect the privacy of subjects by allowing them to refuse to disclose their complete medical history to the investigator

   b. Protect the privacy of investigators by allowing them to refuse to disclose their previous experience as researchers

   c. Protect the privacy of subjects by allowing investigators to refuse to disclose subjects' names or identifying characteristics even if asked to do so by court or governmental agencies

   d. Protect the privacy of sponsors by allowing them to refuse to disclose adverse events unrelated to the study drug

2. A Certificate of Confidentiality prevents disclosure of all but which one of the following:

   a. Substance abuse treatment

   b. Some types of illegal conduct

   c. Names and addresses of subjects

   d. Identifying information voluntarily released by either a subject or an investigator

Chapter 8-11

Training Institutional Review Board Members

1. To participate effectively in IRB review at a minimum, all IRB members should have a core understanding of

   a. 45 CFR 46

   b. Basic ethical principles, regulatory requirements, and the mechanics of serving on an IRB

   c. ICH Guidelines to Good Clinical Practice

   d. OPRR Compliance Activities: Common Findings & Guidance

2. Which IRB members should have more specialized training beyond that of experienced IRB members?

   a. IRB chair, vice-chair, all MDs

   b. Community member(s), new members (less than 6 months on the committee)

   c. IRB chair, vice-chair, legal specialists, advocates for populations served by the IRB

   d. IRB chair, vice-chair, community member(s)

3. Choose the most accurate statement:

   a. New IRB members should only read *The Belmont Report* and the Nuremberg Code before conducting human subject research reviews.

   b. IRB members receive adequate training at IRB meetings.

   c. Only FDA regulations require an IRB to be sufficiently qualified through the experience and expertise of its members.

   d. IRB members should have in-depth knowledge of the history and ethics of human subject protection, regulations governing research in human subjects, and adequate training resources to acquire the knowledge.

Chapter 8-12

Investigator Training

1. According to the authors, the most accurate statement regarding investigator training is

   a. DHHS regulations require sponsors to select qualified investigators and provide them with the information needed to conduct the study properly.

   b. Investigators must be qualified to conduct a research study, uphold the *Belmont* principles and ensure compliance with the regulations and requirements of the IRB.

   c. Education is the most effective method for changing physician behavior.

   d. Investigators who have conducted research in the past do not need any further educational training regarding human subject protection.

2. According to the authors, several effective methods are available to change the behavior of an investigator when designing a training program. Choose the answer that best reflects the three most effective means of influencing investigator behavior:

   a. Education, compliance with federal regulations, performance feedback

   b. Performance feedback, education, administrative rules

   c. Performance feedback, rewards and penalties, participation in improving the process

   d. Administrative rules, rewards and penalties, compliance with federal regulations

3. According to the authors, the answer that best describes one of the four main objectives investigators will master through proper training:

   a. Investigators will understand that the primary goal is the execution of the protocol rather than the protection of their subjects.

   b. Investigators are the only individuals on the research team that have to understand and act according to the ethical principles governing research.

   c. Investigators have to comply only with state and local regulations.

   d. Investigators should understand and apply the *Belmont* principles in research.

4. According to the authors, the answer that best describes the process associated with the successful implementation of an investigator-training program:

   a. An explanation of the direction of the training program and the reasons for its creation; who will be involved and what options investigators have in the training; how the training will be conducted and in what time frame.

   b. The institution establishes a web-based training program and mandates that all investigators participate.

   c. Investigators are allowed to complete the training program when they find the time.

   d. Investigators receive initial communication about the training program and are then responsible for completing it.

Chapter 8-13

Accreditation of Human Research Protection Programs

1. Accreditation is currently being performed by

    a. AAHRPP (Association for the Accreditation of Human Research Protection Programs)

    b. PRIM&R (Public Responsibility in Medicine and Research) and ARENA (Applied Research Ethics National Association)

    c. JCAHO (Joint Commission on Accreditation of Healthcare Organizations) and PRIM&R

    d. AAMC (Association of American Medical Colleges) and ARENA

2. Accreditation of a human research protection program includes

    a. Assessment of IRBs only

    b. Different assessments by the different accrediting bodies

    c. Site visit by a staff member from the accrediting body

    d. Public announcement of results

3. Choose the answer that most accurately describes performance standards used in the accreditation process:

    a. The accreditation process allows the site to choose performance standards that fit its situation.

    b. The accreditation process uses performance standards both in self-assessment and peer review.

    c. The accreditation process requires performance standards to be revised every 3 years.

    d. The accreditation process has different performance standards for biomedical research institutions and social science institutions.

Chapter 8-14

Certification of Institutional Review Board Professionals

1. Certification of IRB professionals is

    a. A professional designation

    b. Legally mandated for IRB staff

    c. A license issued by OHRP

    d. Certificate issued by state agencies

2. Certification helps to raise competency

    a. By having people take a test

    b. By proving understanding of test questions

    c. Through education and training for initial testing and recertification

    d. Through public education programs

3. Preparation for a certification exam should begin by

    a. Reviewing basic regulatory documents and federal guidance

    b. Asking people who have taken the test about the test questions

    c. Reviewing your institution's IRB policy and procedure manual

    d. Reviewing applicable state law

4. Certification is formal recognition that an individual

    a. Can perform a particular job

    b. Is recommended by the certifying body

    c. Should receive a promotion

    d. Has met standards of experience and knowledge

5. The certification program helps raise national standards by

    a. Recognizing federal guidance standards

    b. Creating a "body of knowledge" for the profession

    c. Revising institutional policy and procedure manuals

    d. Harmonizing applicable regulatory documents

Chapter 8-15

Preparing for a Food and Drug Administration Audit

1. The most important document the FDA will review when conducting an IRB audit is

    a. A completed Form 1572 for each investigator

    b. A completed FDA IRB self-audit guide

    c. The IRB written procedures

    d. The institutional assurance for the protection of human research subjects

2. According to the author, to keep track of the conduct of an FDA site visit, it is a good idea to ask the auditor for a brief update

    a. At the completion of the audit

    b. Never, as it will make them suspicious

    c. Only when the auditor requests information

    d. At the end of each audit day

3. The document sent by the FDA to institutions/investigators after an audit that cites serious regulatory deficiencies and demands correction is called

    a. A warning letter

    b. The establishment inspection report

    c. A voluntary action letter

    d. FDA Form 1572

4. A description of the FDA Compliance Program is

    a. A top-secret government document

    b. Available on the web or by writing to the FDA

    c. Available for a small fee only through the Government Printing Office

    d. Included in the FDA Information Sheets

5. Preparation for an FDA audit is best accomplished by the IRB

    a. Through routine self-audits and reviews of IRB procedures and regulatory findings

    b. Between the time the IRB is notified of the audit and when it is conducted

    c. Through an annual review of the IRB minutes

    d. In concert with the FDA reviewers as the audit is being conducted

6. If an IRB receives a Form 483 after an FDA audit

   a. It may not respond until an establishment inspection report is received.

   b. It should respond immediately by phone, requesting clarification of all deficiencies.

   c. It should respond within 7 to 10 days in writing, addressing deficiencies.

   d. A response is required, but only for those deficiencies that the IRB deems have been correctly cited by the FDA.

7. The establishment inspection report (EIR) is produced by

   a. FDA headquarters

   b. The district office

   c. Institutional official

   d. FDA center director

Chapter 8-16

Preparing for an Office for Human Research Protections Site Visit

1. The OHRP's three *statutory* responsibilities are

    a. IRB registration, administration of assurances, and compliance oversight

    b. Coordination of the federal policy (Common Rule), IRB registration, and quality assurance

    c. Technical assistance, education, and quality improvement

    d. Education, administration of assurances, and compliance oversight

2. Most OHRP compliance oversight investigations are resolved:

    a. Through an exchange of correspondence and review of materials and records

    b. After an onsite visit to the relevant institution by OHRP personnel

    c. Without the need for corrective actions

    d. Without formal OHRP determinations

3. The best strategy in preparing for an OHRP compliance site visit is to

    a. Conduct "practice" interviews of IRB members and research investigators.

    b. Invest in long-term prevention through a well-resourced institutional human subject protection program.

    c. Shred any documents that the regulations do not require.

    d. Request that all interviews be conducted in the presence of institutional counsel.

4. After receiving a request to provide OHRP with a report on alleged noncompliance, the institution should

    a. Respond to OHRP as quickly as possible by limiting its review to the specific allegation under investigation.

    b. Impose a "gag order" on the investigator and try to reach an out-of-court settlement with the complainant.

    c. Investigate the alleged noncompliance as thoroughly as possible and, where appropriate, develop an individual or systemic corrective action plan.

    d. Consult outside experts only as a "last resort" and only where proprietary information is not involved.

5. OHRP determination letters are

   a. Considered confidential and protected from release to the public

   b. Available to the public and posted on the OHRP website

   c. Withheld from the press for 30 days after issuance

   d. Shared only with other agencies of the United States Government

6. OHRP takes compliance oversight action

   a. Primarily for punitive purposes, to teach investigators a lesson

   b. To provide other institutions with an example of the dire consequences of a shutdown

   c. To fulfill an annual quota set by OHRP's congressional oversight committees

   d. To ensure present and future protections for human subjects at the institution under scrutiny

7. OHRP's Quality Improvement Program

   a. Is intended to help institutions evaluate and improve the quality of their human research protection program

   b. Is often mandated as a required corrective action after an OHRP determination of noncompliance

   c. Begins with a "blind review" of the institution's human research program by a neutral third party

   d. Was recently terminated by the Office of Management and Budget

8. An "onsite consultation" by OHRP

   a. Indicates that OHRP believes it has evidence of noncompliance

   b. Lasts 3 to 5 days and includes at least two outside experts

   c. Includes attorneys from DHHS and the institution under review

   d. May be requested by an institution following its "Guided Self Assessment"

ANSWER KEY FOR PART 8

Answer Key: Chapter 8-1

1. c
2. b
3. d

Answer Key: Chapter 8-2

1. a
2. d
3. d
4. d

Answer Key: Chapter 8-3

1. c
2. b
3. d
4. b
5. a
6. d
7. c

Answer Key: Chapter 8-4

1. c
2. a
3. c
4. c
5. d

Answer Key: Chapter 8-5

1. d
2. d
3. d
4. d

Answer Key: Chapter 8-6

1. b
2. c

Answer Key: Chapter 8-7

1. b
2. c
3. b
4. c

5. c
6. c
7. b
8. b

Answer Key: Chapter 8-8

1. b
2. b
3. c
4. c

Answer Key: Chapter 8-9

1. a
2. a
3. d
4. b

Answer Key: Chapter 8-10

1. c
2. d

Answer Key: Chapter 8-11

1. b
2. c
3. d

Answer Key: Chapter 8-12

1. b
2. c
3. d
4. a

Answer Key: Chapter 8-13

1. a
2. b
3. b

Answer Key: Chapter 8-14

1. a
2. c
3. a
4. d
5. b

Answer Key: Chapter 8-15

1. c
2. d
3. a
4. b
5. a
6. c
7. b

Answer Key: Chapter 8-16

1. d
2. a
3. b
4. c
5. b
6. d
7. a
8. d

Part 9

Issues Based on Study Population

Chapter 9-1

Vulnerability in Research

1. Which answer best describes what ethicists and regulators usually mean in calling a research population "vulnerable"?

    a. The subjects will be exposed to more significant risks than most other subjects.

    b. The subjects belong to a group that has been stigmatized more than other subjects.

    c. The subjects are less able to protect their own interests than most other subjects.

    d. The subjects have not been provided with as much information as most other subjects.

2. According to current regulations, when an IRB regularly reviews research that involves a vulnerable group of subjects, then it should

    a. Consider requiring investigators to assess decision-making capacity during the consent process

    b. Consider having a consent auditor present during the informed consent process

    c. Consider whether the benefits to society justify the risks to subjects

    d. Consider including on the IRB one or more individual(s) who are knowledgeable about and experienced working with the group of subjects

3. Which is a correct list of the kinds of vulnerability identified by the National Bioethics Advisory Committee?

    a. Cognitive or communicative; institutional; deferential; medical; economic; social

    b. Cognitive or communicative; voluntary; emotional; physical; legal; economic

    c. Minimal; greater than minimal; slightly greater than minimal

    d. Being a woman, a fetus, a neonate, a child, or a prisoner

4. Which of the following vulnerable groups currently has specific regulatory protections?

    a. People with mental disorders

    b. People who are imprisoned

    c. People who cannot read at an 8th grade level

    d. People who desperately need medical treatment

Chapter 9-2

Research in Public Schools

1. School-based research requires the consent of only one parent when

   a. The research involves more than minimal risk.

   b. The research involves no more than minimal risk and there is the prospect of direct benefit to the minor subject.

   c. The research involves more than minimal risk, but may yield generalizable knowledge about the child's disorder or condition.

   d. The research involves more than minimal risk but may present an opportunity to understand, prevent, or alleviate a serious problem affecting the health or welfare of children.

2. Which of the following research activities conducted in public schools may qualify for exemption:

   a. One-on-one interviews with children of divorced families to develop strategies to helping children cope with divorce

   b. Analysis of test data recorded with identifiers to evaluate the effectiveness of a new instructional technique

   c. Research on the effectiveness of a new instructional technique involving the observation of student class participation

   d. Written survey about risky behaviors of middle school children

3. Which of the following research risks are unique to school-based research?

   a. Loss of confidentiality

   b. Peer pressure

   c. Harm to reputation

   d. Peer contagion leading to the reinforcement of negative behavior

4. According to the author, an ethical strategy for increasing student participation in a research study is to

   a. Have the school principal send out the invitation to participate in the research study

   b. Notify students of the number of their peers who have chosen to participate in the study

   c. Send home permission forms with each child

   d. Require faculty to encourage students to return permission forms

Chapter 9-3

Phase I Clinical Trials in Healthy Adults

1. The primary purpose of Phase I clinical trials is

    a. To assess safety

    b. To assess efficacy

    c. To assess compound uniformity

    d. To assess food effect

2. Phase I clinical trials in healthy adults administer doses

    a. Hundreds of times higher than doses tested in animals

    b. Hundreds of times lower than doses tested in animals

    c. That have never been tested in animals

    d. Equivalent to doses tested only in primates

3. Healthy volunteers in a Phase I clinical trial are confined to a research unit because

    a. Being on site is a great way to make friends

    b. Being on site is more profitable for the sponsor

    c. Being on site allows staff to monitor their health and collect biological samples at frequent time points

    d. Being on site enhances their appreciation for the research

4. IRBs should approve stipend amounts in Phase I clinical trials based on

    a. Potential risk

    b. The price of gas

    c. Income levels of volunteers

    d. Time and inconvenience

Chapter 9-4

Requiring Birth Control to Participate in Research

1. The 1994 National Institutes of Health "Guidelines on Inclusion of Women and Minorities as Subjects in Clinical Research" required that women be included in all National Institutes of Health–supported biomedical and behavioral research projects involving human subjects unless a clear and compelling rationale and justification establishes that inclusion is inappropriate. In which of the following cases would it likely be justifiable to exclude (nonpregnant) women?

   a. A study of a new antihypertensive drug, which has not been studied adequately in animals regarding its potential for causing birth defects in pregnant animals

   b. A study of a new antibiotic that is shown to induce mammary tumors in female rats

   c. A study of the comparative effectiveness of two drugs for treatment of acne, for which the investigators are concerned that women will be less compliant in following the complicated drug administration schedule

   d. A study of the comparative effectiveness of two drugs to treat prostate cancer

2. With regard to the use of contraception for women participating in clinical research, which of the following is true?

   a. Exclusion of abstinence as an effective method of birth control is reasonable because it is unlikely to be effective in any population of female subjects.

   b. Barrier methods of contraception are likely to be effective in all populations.

   c. The use of hormonal contraception may compromise drug studies by potentially interfering with the agent under consideration.

   d. The same method of contraception is likely to have the same degree of efficacy for all populations.

3. In its 1994 report on "Ethical and Legal Issues Related to Inclusion of Women in Clinical Studies," the Institute of Medicine recommended all of the following EXCEPT

   a. Women should be enrolled as participants in clinical studies in a manner that ensures that research yields scientifically generalizable results.

   b. The informed consent process should include information regarding the risk of failure of various forms of birth control.

   c. The contraceptive methods to be used should be chosen by the investigator to absolutely minimize the risk to the fetus.

   d. Pregnancy termination options should be discussed as part of the consent process in clinical studies that pose unknown or foreseeable risks to potential offspring.

Chapter 9-5

Research Involving Fetuses and In Vitro Fertilization

1. Choose the statement that most accurately describes the 1996 Dickey-Wicker amendment to the Department of Health and Human Services (DHHS) Budget Bill:

   a. Federal funding may be used for research in which human embryos are destroyed as long as the importance of the research to society is considered to be significant.

   b. This regulation prohibits federal funding of research in which a human embryo is destroyed, discarded, or knowingly subjected to risk greater than that allowed for research on fetuses in utero.

   c. Federal funding may be used for research in which human embryos are destroyed as long as they were going to be destroyed for reasons other than the research.

   d. This regulation prohibits federal funding of research in which a human embryo is subjected to more than minimal risk of surviving with a genetic mutation.

2. Choose the most accurate statement regarding federal regulations related to research involving fetuses:

   a. Federal regulations prohibit monetary or other inducements to fetal tissue donors.

   b. Federal regulations require that research directors control the timing and method used to terminate a pregnancy.

   c. Federal regulations permit research procedures that are likely to cause fetal death in situations where the importance of the research to society is high.

   d. Federal regulations encourage research participants to require that donated fetal tissue be used only for a close relative who is in need of a fetal tissue transplant.

3. Choose the answer that most accurately describes the situations in which federal regulations permit the IRB to approve research that is directed at the fetus itself:

   a. Whenever the risk of research participation for the mother is no more than minimal

   b. Whenever both the biologic mother and father of the fetus give informed consent

   c. When the mother agrees that the risk/benefit profile of the research for the fetus is favorable

   d. When the purpose of the research is to address the health needs of a particular fetus or the risk of the research to the fetus is minimal, and the purpose of the research is to develop important knowledge that cannot be obtained by other means

4. Which of the following is a problem associated with current U.S. federal policy on stem cell lines:

   a. There are too many cell lines available for federally funded research, forcing a choice of which cell lines should be used.

   b. Many of the federally funded cell lines are from frozen embryos.

   c. There are only 22 such lines, and all are contaminated with molecules derived from the mouse cell feeder layers on which they were cultured.

   d. The original embryo donors expect to use these cell lines for their own medical benefit.

Chapter 9-6

Research Involving Pregnant Women

1. Choose the most accurate statement:

   a. In 1993, FDA regulations were revised to emphasize that it is considered unethical to routinely exclude women of childbearing potential from research involving investigational medications.

   b. FDA regulations currently prohibit research involving an investigational medication in women of childbearing potential.

   c. Federal regulations require IRBs to use the same criteria for approving research involving women of childbearing potential as for women who are known to be pregnant.

   d. Federal regulations state that abstinence is not an effective way to avoid an unwanted pregnancy.

2. Choose the most accurate statement:

   a. When a high likelihood of teratogenicity justifies exclusion of women of childbearing potential from research, the protocol should require restrictions on male subjects that recognize the potential risk to fertile sexual partners.

   b. The author of this chapter reminds the IRB that it is important to test drugs that are highly teratogenic in pregnant women.

   c. Federal regulations require two simultaneous forms of birth control for a woman of childbearing potential to participate in research involving an investigational medication.

   d. Federal regulations require that Phase I drug testing be limited to women of childbearing potential.

3. Choose the most accurate statement:

   a. There is no situation in which current DHHS regulations permit a pregnant woman to participate in research when the risk to the fetus is more than minimal.

   b. In March 2001, DHHS regulations became effective that required paternal consent to enroll a pregnant woman in research.

   c. In March 2001, DHHS regulations became effective that promote a policy of inclusion for pregnant women in research.

   d. Federal regulations permit payments or other inducements to terminate a pregnancy during research under certain well-defined situations.

Chapter 9-7

Research Involving Children

1. In *The Belmont Report*, the "special provisions" for children that respect for persons requires include

    a. The opportunity to choose to the extent they are able, honoring dissent, and seeking the permission of other parties to protect the subjects from harm

    b. The opportunity to choose to the extent they are able and seeking the permission of other parties to protect the subjects from harm

    c. The opportunity to choose to the extent they are able and honoring dissent

    d. Honoring dissent and seeking the permission of other parties to protect the subjects from harm

2. What concepts form the basis for the "special protection" of children?

    a. Minimal risk, prospect of direct benefit, IRB approval, and assent

    b. Minimal risk, prospect of direct benefit, assent, and permission

    c. Minimal risk, IRB approval, assent, and permission

    d. Minimal risk, prospect of direct benefit, and permission

3. Which of the following statements is correct regarding research that can be considered exempt from further IRB review?

    a. There are no special conditions for exempt review for children. IRBs should follow current regulations for exempt reviews.

    b. The research involves only the observation of public behavior when the investigator(s) participates in the activities being observed.

    c. Survey and interview research with children cannot be considered exempt.

    d. Educational testing of children can be considered exempt.

4. The IRB can approve research involving children only if it falls into one of three categories, provided that all of the criteria found in 45 CFR 46.111 are also fulfilled. Which of the following statements is not one of the approved categories?

    a. Research involving an intervention or procedure presenting more than minimal risk to children that offers the "prospect of direct benefit" or may "contribute to the well-being" of the individual child

    b. Research presenting "no greater than minimal risk to children"

    c. Research involving an intervention or procedure that presents only a "minor increase over minimal risk" yet does not offer any "prospect of direct benefit" or "contribute to the well-being" of the child

    d. Research involving an intervention or procedure presenting more than minimal risk to children that offers the "prospect of direct benefit" or may "contribute to the well-being" of the individual child or their family

5. Choose the correct statement. In evaluating whether a given procedure or intervention qualifies as "minimal risk," an IRB should consider

   a. Whether the risks presented are less than the risks that parents may ordinarily allow their children to experience in the course of their everyday lives

   b. Whether the risks presented are comparable to the risks that parents may ordinarily allow their children to experience in the course of their everyday lives

   c. Whether the risks presented are greater than the risks that parents may ordinarily allow their children to experience in the course of their everyday lives

   d. Whether the risks presented are comparable to the risks the researchers feel the children experience in the course of their everyday lives

6. Parental or guardian permission is treated in much the same way as informed consent, apart from some additional provisions found in §46.408. Choose the correct statement that describes these provisions:

   a. Both parents must give permission for research approved under §46.408.

   b. Both parents must give permission for research approved under §46.408 unless one parent is not reasonably available.

   c. Parental permission may be waived as not being a reasonable requirement to protect a child to allow access to an FDA-regulated product.

   d. If a child is judged by the investigator to be capable of assent, parental permission may be waived.

7. Choose the correct statement about child assent:

   a. An investigator can assume that a child has assented to research participation as long as the child does not voice an objection.

   b. An investigator can assume that a child has assented to research participation as long as the child does not voice an objection, provided that the parent agrees with this assessment.

   c. Assent can be waived if the parent thinks that the purpose of the research is sufficiently important.

   d. If a child is capable of assent, assent to participation in more than minimal-risk research can be waived only if the child may directly benefit from a research intervention that is not otherwise available outside the research.

Chapter 9-8

Research Involving Adults with Decisional Impairment

1. Adults with decisional impairment should not be involved in studies that could otherwise be conducted with capable subjects unless

   a. They are included as a control population.

   b. They may benefit from study participation.

   c. Safety is first established in subjects with capacity.

   d. The lack of capacity is a temporary condition.

2. According to the author, the signature of the person assessing the capacity of a potential subject attests to

   a. The subject's capacity to consent at that time

   b. The subject's capacity throughout the duration of the study

   c. The need for caregiver consent at some point during the study

   d. The subject's complete understanding of study procedures

3. Asking a study subject to appoint a surrogate is advised

   a. When the research involves complex procedures and more than minimal risk

   b. In accordance with applicable federal regulations

   c. When the subject is enrolled in a study involving greater than minimal risk

   d. If it is anticipated that the subject may lose capacity during the study

4. The subject's ability to evidence a choice is a standard of capacity that reflects the ability to

   a. Communicate a "yes or no" decision

   b. Understand relevant information

   c. Appreciate a situation and its likely consequences

   d. Manipulate information rationally

5. The appointment of a surrogate to consent for research involving an incapable subject

   a. Is specifically addressed in federal regulations

   b. Is a matter of state law and varies from state to state

   c. Is equivalent to the appointment of a surrogate to treatment

   d. Requires approval by a court to be valid

6. Consent by a family member for a subject who lacks capacity is generally accepted

   a. For research involving greater than minimal risk and no possibility of benefit

   b. For studies involving emergency room interventions

   c. For research that poses minimal risk or the possibility of benefit

   d. For studies involving a minor increase over minimal risk

Chapter 9-9

Regulatory Issues of Research Involving Prisoners

1. Which of the following provides additional specific protections pertaining to biomedical and behavioral research involving prisoners as subjects?

   a. 45 CFR 46, Subpart A

   b. 45 CFR 46, Subpart B

   c. 45 CFR 46, Subpart C

   d. 45 CFR 46, Subpart D

2. Although all may be vulnerable individuals who should be afforded additional protections, which of the following persons in the circumstance described is a prisoner according to the definition provided in 45 CFR 46.303(c)?

   a. An individual who has been released from the city jail and is out on bail

   b. An individual who is arrested and released on his or her own recognizance

   c. An individual who has been paroled from a federal prison

   d. An individual detained in a county penal institution pending arraignment

3. Choose the most accurate statement regarding the requirement for the presence of a prisoner or prisoner representative in order for the full IRB to review research involving prisoners:

   a. Only required for initial review

   b. Only required for initial and continuing review

   c. Only required for initial review, continuing review, and protocol amendments

   d. Required for initial review, continuing review, protocol amendments, and review of adverse events

4. Which of the following DHHS-funded research with prisoners can be independently reviewed and approved by an IRB under DHHS regulations at 45 CFR 46.306?

   a. Research concerning the process of incarceration

   b. Research on hepatitis C infection

   c. Research involving a placebo control

   d. Research involving an HIV vaccine

5. What is the only subject population that has additional protections requiring certification by Office for Human Research Protections (OHRP) before IRB approval of DHHS-funded research?

    a. Pregnant women

    b. Older persons

    c. Prisoners

    d. Mentally incompetent

6. When a research subject is both a prisoner and a minor, what sections of 45 CFR 46 must be taken into consideration:

    a. Only Subpart C

    b. Only Subpart D

    c. Both Subparts C and D

    d. Neither Subpart D or C

Chapter 9-10

Research Involving College Students

1. How can an IRB help insure that research participation for course credit is not coercive?

   a. The IRB should not allow research participation as a course requirement.

   b. The IRB should understand the structure of the course requirement to make sure that there is an alternative option to fulfill the requirement.

   c. The IRB should interview participants in research to make sure they do not feel as if they were forced to participate.

   d. The IRB is not responsible for ensuring that research participation is not coercive.

2. A student makes a complaint to the IRB that they were forced to participate in research studies because their class required it. The IRB should

   a. Take immediate action to temporarily suspend the study until further notice.

   b. Determine whether there was an alternative assignment that the student could complete for the course that was comparable in scope to the study.

   c. Reprimand the course professor for imposing the requirement.

   d. Do nothing. It is not the role of the IRB to micromanage participant complaints.

3. Which of the following is NOT a concern when the IRB reviews research studies that plan to recruit college students?

   a. Whether any of the participants are under the age of 18 years

   b. Whether the level of incentive offered is extreme

   c. Whether the study includes both genders

   d. Whether the participant can withdraw from the study at any point

ANSWER KEY FOR PART 9

Answer Key: Chapter 9-1
1. c
2. d
3. a
4. b

Answer Key: Chapter 9-2
1. b
2. c
3. d
4. d

Answer Key: Chapter 9-3
1 a
2 b
3 c
4 d

Answer Key: Chapter 9-4
1. d
2. c
3. c

Answer Key: Chapter 9-5
1. b
2. a
3. d
4. c

Answer Key: Chapter 9-6
1. a
2. a
3. c

Answer Key: Chapter 9-7
1. a
2. b
3. c
4. d
5. b
6. b
7. d

Answer Key: Chapter 9-8
1. b
2. a
3. d
4. a
5. b
6. c

Answer Key: Chapter 9-9
1. c
2. d
3. d
4. a
5. c
6. c

Answer Key: Chapter 9-10
1. b
2. b
3. c

Part 10

IRB Issues Based on Study Design or Category

Chapter 10-1

When Are Research Risks Reasonable in Relationship to Anticipated Benefits?

1. The standard of clinical equipoise is satisfied when

   a. The institutional review board (IRB) has determined that participation in a trial would provide therapeutic benefit to the research subject.

   b. The IRB has determined that experts would disagree about the preferable course of treatment.

   c. The IRB has determined that the risks are equal to the benefits of the research.

   d. The IRB has determined that the risks of participation in a clinical trial are minimized.

2. According to the authors, research risks are reasonable when

   a. Therapeutic procedures meet the standards of clinical equipoise, and nontherapeutic procedures offer direct benefit to research subjects.

   b. Therapeutic procedures offer direct benefit to research subjects, and nontherapeutic procedures meet the standards of clinical equipoise.

   c. Therapeutic procedures meet the standards of clinical equipoise, and nontherapeutic procedures pose risks that are minimized and reasonable in light of the knowledge to be gained.

   d. Therapeutic procedures are likely to lead to generalizable results, and nontherapeutic procedures are consistent with sound, scientific design.

3. Which of the following statements most accurately explains the value of component analysis, according to the authors?

   a. Component analysis is useful for analyzing clinical research studies involving placebo controls or incapable adults.

   b. Component analysis presents a systematic approach to analyzing the ethical issues of a research protocol involving therapeutic procedures.

   c. Component analysis provides clear criteria to IRBs assessing the ethics of clinical research involving both therapeutic and non-therapeutic procedures, which leads to consistent decision making and enables principled resolution of contemporary controversies.

   d. Component analysis provides accurate ethical guidance for making sound judgments about the ethics of clinical research.

Chapter 10-2

Internet Research: A Brief Guide for Institutional Review Boards

1. According to the author, what are the two sources of potential harm to subjects from participating in Internet research activities?

   a. Loss of employment and damage to reputation

   b. Loss of dignity and privacy

   c. Adverse psychological reactions resulting from participation in the research and breach of confidentiality

   d. Physical and emotional harm

2. According to the author, for research posing minimal risk to participants, electronic informed consent may be possible as follows:

   a. Participants are presented with electronic information about the research study. Access to the study is not allowed until the participant has clicked a button that says "I accept" to express consent to participation.

   b. The participant is e-mailed informed consent documentation that he or she downloads, reviews, signs, and returns to the researcher by regular mail.

   c. The researcher e-mails informed consent documentation and assumes that the participant has consented by his or her participation in the research.

   d. Electronic informed consent is never possible.

3. According to the author, an effective way to protect the confidentiality of sensitive data is to

   a. Create anonymous online identities

   b. Employ third-party software that "strips" data of all identifiers

   c. Transmit data using personal e-mail

   d. Transmit data to private listserv

Chapter 10-3

Qualitative Social Science Research

1. Professor Jolly, a sociologist at a prestigious university, has received federal funding for a one-time survey of several hundred young adults who are graduates of an after-school music education program for inner-city children. School authorities believe that individuals who participated in the program are less likely to abuse drugs or run afoul of the law and more likely to succeed in college. The local economy is struggling, and the state legislature feels mounting pressure from a taxpayers' organization to cut "nonessential" programs. If the research does not demonstrate that the program is clearly effective, funding may be reduced or eliminated.

   Which one of the following recommendations *would be most appropriate* for the IRB reviewing this study to issue?

   a. Professor Jolly should not ask his subjects any questions about prior drug use or legal troubles because such information could be vulnerable to subpoena.

   b. Professor Jolly must obtain informed consent from *current* program participants. Even though they are not subjects in this study, if the program funding is cut, their lives will be affected.

   c. Professor Jolly should not link his subjects' identities to their responses because they will be discussing potentially stigmatizing aspects of their own behavior.

   d. Professor Jolly may need to discard some data if preliminary results do not indicate that the program has a beneficial effect in order to ensure that the program funding continues.

2. Which of the following statements is correct?

   a. Social science researchers' data, as is the case with lawyers' and clergies' communications, enjoy protection from subpoena if the researcher has promised confidentiality to subjects.

   b. Most risks in qualitative social science research occur during interaction with subjects. After subject participation is complete, the risk of harm drops effectively to zero.

   c. A certificate of confidentiality will provide protection against forced disclosure of data, but only when the research is federally funded.

   d. IRBs may consider the benefits to society of applying knowledge gained from the research when weighing risks and benefits of a proposed research project.

3. Ms. Clean, a graduate student in education, wants to interview elementary school children about their relationships with classmates, siblings, and parents. She hypothesizes that children who "act out" and are dominant in the classroom will be similarly dominant at home. Several of her open-ended questions deal with physical as well as social aggression. At the IRB meeting, members express some concerns about the study.

   Which one of the following recommendations *would be most appropriate* for the IRB reviewing this study to issue?

a. Because a child could reveal details of an abuse or neglect situation, Ms. Clean must obtain a Certificate of Confidentiality so that she will not be required to report such a situation to authorities.

b. Because Ms. Clean is asking children to describe situations in which they are physically dominant or aggressive, she should be careful not to imply approval of those behaviors.

c. Ms. Clean should remove any questions that deal with physical as well as social aggression.

d. If Ms. Clean will provide a copy of her findings to teachers and parents, she need not disguise her subjects' identities beyond removing their names from the data because teachers and parents know the subjects already.

4. Which of the following statements is correct?

a. The IRB is not responsible for eliminating risk from a research protocol as part of its review and approval process.

b. An investigator is prohibited from voluntarily revealing identifiable information about a research subject if he or she has obtained a Certificate of Confidentiality.

c. Qualitative social science research, because it presents little risk of harm, is always either exempt or eligible for expedited IRB review.

d. By definition, behavior in a public setting is subject to observation by others, and thus, it cannot be considered "private."

5. What method does the author suggest for ensuring that subjects are truly informed of the risks and benefits of participation in qualitative research when all of the risks cannot be anticipated?

a. To draft a consent document that identifies all possible risks of participation

b. To include a statement in the informed consent document that informs subjects that not all risks of participation can be identified

c. To provide ongoing information to subjects of the risks and benefits of participation as new data are acquired

d. To include a statement in the informed consent document that assures subjects that all risks are minimal

Chapter 10-4

Ethnographic Research

1. In general, which phase of the research process introduces the greatest potential risk to participants involved in participant observation?

   a. Recruitment

   b. Obtaining informed consent

   c. Data collection

   d. Termination/dissemination of data

2. In general, researchers planning studies involving ethnographic methods should be expected to

   a. Obtain written consent from every person with whom they interact during the scope of the project

   b. Avoid recording identifying information if possible

   c. Ask the IRB for blanket approval of a general research idea and then work out the specific details once fieldwork has begun

   d. Provide participants with a specific list of topics that will and will not be addressed during the course of the study

3. A researcher contacts the IRB regarding planned research involving participant observation of children in a special need preschool. The researcher has obtained the written permission of the school's director. Information that could potentially identify the participants will not be recorded and the details identifying the research site will be obscured in all publications. The study

   a. Should not be submitted to the IRB

   b. Should be designated as exempt from further IRB review provided that the IRB does not identify any additional risks

   c. Could receive expedited review provided that the IRB has not identified any additional risks

   d. Must receive full committee review

4. A graduate-level researcher wishes to study the influence of familial pressure on academic performance among teenagers in a school setting in Taiwan. She has obtained school permission to conduct the research and requests a waiver of parental permission. The IRB is unsure about Taiwanese customs in this area. The IRB should

   a. Trust the researcher's expertise in the research setting and grant the waiver.

   b. Refuse to grant the waiver. It's better to be safe than sorry.

   c. Identify an uninvolved expert in this field setting to serve as a consultant to the IRB.

   d. Let the school director decide whether the waiver is appropriate.

5. A researcher wishes to conduct ethnographic research in a Buddhist monastery. Interviews will be recorded without identifiers and documentation of informed consent will be waived. The researcher will store the audio tapes in a locked box in his possession indefinitely. Names and other identifying information will not be included in any reports of the data. Which of the following statements should be included in the consent script?

a. Participation in this study is anonymous.

b. Participation in this study is confidential.

c. Participation in this study is anonymous and confidential.

d. Participation in this study is neither anonymous nor confidential.

Chapter 10-5

Health Services Research

1. IRBs often have trouble evaluating and monitoring projects that involve health services research because

   a. Federal regulations imply that all health services research is exempt from IRB review.

   b. Federal regulations hold health services research to different standards than other kinds of research.

   c. All health services research involves subjects from countries other than the United States.

   d. Health services research usually focuses on groups or systems rather than individuals.

2. Some individuals feel that federal regulations are currently not applicable to many health services research projects because

   a. Health services research may involve multisite research.

   b. In health services research, the true subject—the entity who is the focus of the research—is often a group or organization rather than the individual whose health information is being recorded.

   c. Federal regulations are biased against social science research.

   d. Federal regulations do not direct the IRB to evaluate issues related to privacy and confidentiality.

3. Which statement best describes the difference between the "true social experiment" and the "natural experiment?"

   a. The true social experiment involves the voluntary enrollment of people into randomized experimental models of organizational systems, whereas the natural experiment examines data that occur naturally following major practice or policy changes in the health care system.

   b. The true social experiment involves the voluntary enrollment of people into randomized experimental models of organizational systems, whereas the natural experiment allows subjects to choose which arm of the experiment they prefer to be enrolled.

   c. The true social experiment involves the systematic collection of data, whereas the natural experiment involves the analysis of data collected for other purposes.

   d. The true social experiment examines data that occur following major practice or policy changes in the health care system, whereas the natural experiment involves the voluntary enrollment of people into randomized experimental models of organizational systems.

Chapter 10-6

Epidemiology/Public Health Research

1. A public health activity is research under the Department of Health and Human Services (DHHS) definition of research when

   a. The activity is a systematic investigation and is designed to generate new knowledge that will contribute to the scientific literature.

   b. The activity involves scientific methodologies such as epidemiologic or statistical methods without regard to the intention of the activity.

   c. The activity involves human beings.

   d. The activity involves risks such as breaches in maintaining confidentiality of the identifiable data.

2. Risks concerning privacy and confidentiality are often a concern in epidemiologic research. Which statement best describes the nature of these risks?

   a. Privacy and confidentiality are the same concerns. Minimizing the risk of one minimizes the risks of the other.

   b. Privacy and confidentiality are two different concepts and require separate types of protections to minimize risks.

   c. Risks to privacy and confidentiality are the only risks associated with epidemiologic research.

   d. Privacy and confidential risks are always minimal.

3. Epidemiologic research often involves the review of thousands of records and existing data. Investigators often request a waiver of informed consent to review these materials. Select the most appropriate statement concerning the waiver of informed consent for this kind of research:

   a. When existing data are used in an epidemiologic study, the informed consent process can be automatically waived under 45 CFR 46.116 by the IRB.

   b. The IRB must determine that each of the four criteria for waiving informed consent under 45 CFR 46.116 are met before approving a waiver.

   c. The only criteria for waiving informed consent in epidemiologic research under 45 CFR 46.116 are that the research involves only minimal risk and it would be impracticable to carry out the research without the waiver.

   d. The IRB cannot waive the informed consent process in epidemiologic research, but it can waive the requirement for documentation of informed consent.

4. Data collection methods in public health research

    a. Are often the same as those used in public health practice activities

    b. Are used to define whether the activity is research according to the federal definition for protecting human research subjects

    c. Are restricted to surveys and review of records

    d. Are related to whether the information is publishable

Chapter 10-7

Survey Research

1. What is the principal risk posed by survey research?

   a. Physical harm

   b. Privacy/confidentiality

   c. Coercion

   d. Legal claims

2. Why should IRB reviewers care about response rates to surveys?

   a. Low response rates may change the risk/benefit analysis of the study.

   b. It is expensive to increase response rates.

   c. Researchers might miscalculate them.

   d. High response rates increase risk to subjects.

3. Surrogate surveys pose ethical challenges because

   a. Respondents give informed consent.

   b. Parents cannot give consent for their children.

   c. The ultimate target of the survey may not be reachable.

   d. Vulnerable populations are targeted.

4. Choose the payment method that the author suggests will reduce coercion and obtain required response rates:

   a. Payment of $25 after the survey is completed

   b. Payment of $1 to $5 up front

   c. Do not provide payment

   d. Payment of $25 up front

Chapter 10-8

Research Involving a Medical Device

1. What information must an IRB have prior to reviewing a study involving a medical device?

    a. The countries in which it has gained regulatory approval

    b. The studies regarding competing or prior similar devices

    c. The regulatory and investigational status of the device in the United States

    d. The insurance coverage provided by the sponsor

2. What is the net effect on the investigator and sponsor of an IRB decision that a device is a nonsignificant risk (NSR) device?

    a. It means that for continuing review the expedited process can be used.

    b. It means that the Food and Drug Administration (FDA) might not learn about the study until a marketing application is submitted.

    c. It grants the sponsor a 510K for the device.

    d. It means that the FDA must review the study before it can be initiated.

3. An exception from the investigational device exemption (IDE) requirement might best be claimed by the sponsor of

    a. An extremely low-risk device

    b. An in vitro diagnostic device

    c. A study of a Class 1 device

    d. A commercial device used off-label

4. Every IRB policy and procedure regarding devices should have a statement about which topic?

    a. How to make an NSR decision

    b. How to determine substantial equivalence

    c. How to evaluate the classification of the device

    d. When to grant a 510K

5. Which statements are true about humanitarian use devices (HUDs)?

a. 1 and 3

b. 2 and 3

c. 3 and 4

d. 1 and 4

 1. Must be used in a research context

 2. May be sold

 3. Have been cleared by the FDA without information on effectiveness

 4. Are for a condition affecting up to 10,000 patients per year

Chapter 10-9

Humanitarian Use Devices

1. Choose the most accurate statement regarding a HUD:

   a. FDA regulations do not require IRB approval to use a HUD.

   b. FDA regulations require IRB approval to use a HUD.

   c. FDA regulations are silent on the need for IRB approval when using a HUD.

   d. FDA regulations permit the use of a HUD only in a life-threatening medical condition.

2. Choose the most accurate statement regarding a HUD:

   a. Federal regulations state that the use of a HUD is exempt from IRB review when risk is no more than minimal.

   b. Federal regulations require a clinical trial to document efficacy of a HUD.

   c. Federal regulations require IRBs to limit approval of a HUD to a period of 6 months.

   d. Federal regulations require IRB approval even when HUD use does not involve research.

Chapter 10-10

Banking of Human Biological Materials for Research

1. Choose the most accurate statement:

   a. Federal regulations prohibit a "study within a study" consent document in which subjects are asked to donate tissue for research in addition to participating in the primary study.

   b. A consent document for the donation of tissue for research testing should explain the method for withdrawing a specimen from the repository.

   c. Consent documents to donate tissue for research should include a statement that the subjects waive their right to benefit financially from anything resulting from the research activity.

   d. Research that is limited to the testing of tissue specimens associated with identifiers that would otherwise be discarded is always exempt from IRB review.

2. Choose the most accurate statement regarding the donation of tissue for research:

   a. The informed consent process must clarify two main issues: whether the tissue is going to be linked to personal identifiers and whether the tissue will be tested for genetic markers that are known to predict disease.

   b. Federal regulations require that subjects be paid if they donate their tissue for research.

   c. Federal regulations require that subjects be given the results of research tests involving their tissue if they ask for it.

   d. Research on tissue specimens never requires IRB approval because a tissue specimen is not a human subject.

3. Which of the following requires the most attention in terms of an IRB's risk assessment of a proposed repository research activity that requires familial or ethnic DNA/genetic material?

   a. Somatic cell evaluation

   b. Geographic location of tissue collection

   c. Germline cell evaluation

   d. Security of repository

4. Which of the following best describes a key responsibility of the gatekeeper of a research specimen repository?

   a. Denies access to specimens by commercial organizations

   b. Notifies individual subjects or next of kin prior to each release of a contributed stored repository specimen

   c. Confirms access to banked specimens occurs with IRB approval, where applicable

   d. Determines whether a waiver of consent is appropriate

Chapter 10-11

The Placebo-Controlled Clinical Trial

1. Choose the answer that describes the question that is most important for the IRB to ask when evaluating the risk of placebo:

   a. Is the toxicity of standard treatment considered to be high?

   b. Does the problem that the person is being treated for cause severe suffering?

   c. Could the use of placebo instead of standard therapy in this setting cause irreversible health problems?

   d. Does the study provide for "rescue" therapy if subjects do not respond to placebo?

2. Choose the question that is most important when evaluating the need for a study design that involves concomitant placebo control:

   a. Will an active control study require more subjects than a placebo-controlled trial?

   b. Is it possible to predict the placebo response rate in this study with a reasonable degree of accuracy?

   c. Does the study sponsor prefer a placebo-controlled trial?

   d. Does the study involve an investigational medication?

3. Choose the most accurate statement:

   a. Most placebo-controlled trials are designed to test equivalence, not efficacy.

   b. An efficacy trial with placebo control usually requires more subjects than an equivalence trial with an active control.

   c. In an efficacy trial with a placebo control, there is an incentive for quality control that is not present in an equivalence trial with an active control.

   d. Most studies with active treatment control arms are designed to test efficacy, not equivalence.

4. Four medical research trials are described below. Choose the answer that describes the trial where the use of placebo is MOST LIKELY to present ethical problems:

   a. In a trial of an investigational medication in patients with severe heart failure, one group receives best standard treatment plus study drug, and the other receives best standard treatment plus placebo.

   b. A trial randomizes subjects with severe heart failure to either an investigational medication or placebo. Subjects are not permitted to take additional medication during the course of the trial. Patients are eligible for the trial only if they have not responded to any of the standard treatments for their condition.

   c. In a trial of an investigational medication to relieve pain in patients who have had pain for many years from degenerative arthritis of the spine, subjects are randomized between the study medication and placebo. Most eligible subjects will have tried all approved treatments for their pain, but this is not a requirement for research participation.

d. In a trial of an investigational medication to prevent the severe nausea and vomiting that usually follows high-dose chemotherapy for cancer, subjects are randomized to study medication or placebo. The use of additional medication is prohibited during the course of the study. Approved medications are considered to be moderately effective and well tolerated in this setting, but better medications are clearly needed. This study is limited to patients who have not received chemotherapy in the past and thus have no prior experience with nausea medication in this setting.

Chapter 10-12

Treatment-Withholding Studies in Psychiatry

1. When considering studies that involve withholding psychiatric treatment the IRB should

    a. Vote to not approve such studies.

    b. Use caution when the illness in question is likely to cause dangerous behavior.

    c. Appoint a subcommittee.

    d. Vote to approve studies that do not involve anti-psychotic drugs.

2. A factor that should increase the likelihood of IRB approval of studies involving withholding psychiatric treatment is

    a. Exclusion of people over age 60

    b. Exclusion of pregnant women

    c. Provision for timely "rescue" if symptoms worsen

    d. Consent from surrogate decision makers

3. When IRB members are uncertain about the ethical merit of a study involving withholding of a psychiatric drug treatment, it would be wise to

    a. Seek the opinion of a qualified consultant.

    b. Vote to not approve the study.

    c. Vote to exclude patients with depressive symptoms.

    d. Tell the investigator to redesign the study.

4. IRBs might have difficulty evaluating psychiatric treatment withholding studies because

    a. Most psychiatric illness can be cured with currently available drug therapy.

    b. Most psychiatric patients are not capable of giving informed consent.

    c. The dropout rate in psychiatric studies approaches 50%.

    d. The natural history of many psychiatric illnesses is hard to predict.

5. Compelling evidence that schizophrenia causes neuronal injury that could be prevented by drug treatment would

    a. Mean the end of research about schizophrenia

    b. End the need for ethical awareness about psychiatric research

    c. Add weight to arguments against studies that involve withholding drug treatment

    d. Cause IRBs to be overwhelmed with new research proposals

6. IRBs should carefully consider studies involving withholding psychiatric drug treatment because

   a. Such research holds little promise.

   b. Such studies represent an area of research where ethical controversy exists.

   c. Such research is inherently unethical.

   d. No safeguards could possibly protect subjects from significant harm.

Chapter 10-13

Phase I Oncology Trials

1. Choose the most accurate statement:

   a. The classic Phase I oncology study is planned to induce toxicity but has no realistic expectation of direct benefit to research subjects.

   b. The literature shows that about 10% of the subjects who participate in Phase I oncology trials are cured of their disease.

   c. Studies show that the main reason subjects participate in Phase I oncology trials is to help people in the future, not to benefit directly from the drugs they will receive in the study.

   d. There are no alternatives to study design used in the classic Phase I oncology trial.

2. Choose the answer that most accurately describes Benjamin Freedman's summary of the fundamental ethical issue in Phase I oncology trials:

   a. In Phase I oncology trials, subjects read and sign a consent document that accurately describes the trial. They know what they are doing.

   b. Phase I oncology trials are ethical because there is a remote chance that subjects will respond favorably to the study treatment.

   c. Investigators often imply that a Phase I oncology trial is a study of safety and efficacy. Calling a toxicity study a study of safety seems harmless, but calling it a study of efficacy is simply false, although, to be sure, if there were no hope of the drug working, it would not be tested.

   d. It is unethically paternalistic to prevent a desperate cancer patient from participating in a study if there is any chance, regardless of how remote, that he or she will benefit from the study treatment.

3. Choose the answer that most accurately describes the author's view on "therapeutic misconceptions" in Phase I oncology trials:

   a. Therapeutic misconceptions exist because the consent document does not explain the study correctly.

   b. Informed consent is a problem in Phase I oncology trials because both the subjects and physician–investigators share the therapeutic misconception.

   c. The therapeutic misconception applies only to research subjects; physician–investigators clearly understand the goals of the trial and explain this accurately to potential subjects.

   d. The therapeutic misconception is a good thing in oncology research because it is important to give people with cancer as much hope as possible.

4. The last section of this chapter presents recommendations for IRB review of Phase I oncology trials. Choose the answer that most accurately describes the author's recommendations:

    a. The IRB should recognize that the benefits of "close follow-up" or "free medical care" mean that Phase I oncology trials are ethical.

    b. The "risks" section of the consent document should downplay the chance of toxicity.

    c. The consent document should emphasize that a goal of the study is to evaluate efficacy.

    d. The "benefits" section of the consent document should say: "Based on prior experience, the chance that you will feel better or live longer from participating in this study is almost zero."

5. Which statement provides the best explanation for the author's position that intrapatient dose escalation is an acceptable alternative to cohort-specific dosing schedules more commonly employed in Phase I studies?

    a. This approach allows administration of the highest safely achievable dose of the anticancer agent, which typically has the best chance of killing cancer cells.

    b. Intrapatient dose escalation increases the likelihood of therapeutic benefit to research subjects.

    c. Intrapatient dose escalation will yield more meaningful research data.

    d. Intrapatient dose escalation allows the research subject greater autonomy.

Chapter 10-14

Research Involving Genetic Testing

1. The major focus during IRB review of studies with genetic testing should be on

   a. Confidentiality and privacy

   b. Compensation for research-related injury

   c. Physical risks

   d. Payment to participants

2. According to this author, in reviewing genetic studies involving analysis of family pedigrees, one needs to be very careful that there will be no

   a. Coercion of family members

   b. Payment of participants

   c. Conflict of interest

   d. Research-related injury

3. Genetic testing studies must always

   a. Give participants the option of not receiving information.

   b. Destroy all tissue samples after 5 years.

   c. Provide monetary compensation to participants.

   d. Inform participants of the precise nature of the testing.

Chapter 10-15

International Research

1. To receive a federalwide assurance, non-U.S. institutions

   a. Must adopt 45 CFR 46 or commensurate guidelines

   b. Are required to have established an IRB

   c. Must receive funding from the U.S. National Institutes of Health

   d. Must register with the U.S. FDA

2. Knowledge of the local research context should be obtained by the reviewing IRB. The Office for Human Research Protections (OHRP) suggests that the depth of knowledge should be commensurate to

   a. The number of participants expected to enroll in the research

   b. The level of risk that the research entails

   c. The distance between the location of the reviewing IRB and the research site

   d. The professional credentials and research experience of the local investigator

3. DHHS regulations at 45 CFR 46.116 require that information related to informed consent be provided in language that is understandable to the subject. In research settings where the local language is not English, it is advisable that the IRB

   a. Add IRB members who are fluent in the language spoken at the research site

   b. Carefully scrutinize the English-language version

   c. Review a back-translated version of any informed consent materials

   d. Contract with a translation service to provide accurate translations

4. To prevent problems at foreign research sites

   a. IRBs should maintain close communication with research staff in the field.

   b. Members of the reviewing IRB should conduct site-monitoring visits on a regularly scheduled basis.

   c. U.S. IRBs should proactively communicate with host-country IRBs.

   d. IRBs should maintain close communication with OHRP and the FDA.

Chapter 10-16

Alternative Medicine Research

1. Choose the most accurate statement:

   a. The risk of research involving alternative medicine is always minimal.

   b. Most state laws require a medical license to dispense medicinal herbs, such as St. John's wort.

   c. Federal regulations state that research involving alternative medicine is exempt from IRB review.

   d. Many herbs, other botanicals, and mineral and amino acids are not regulated by the FDA because they are considered "dietary supplements" by federal law passed in 1990 and 1994.

2. Choose the most accurate statement:

   a. Federal regulations regarding IRB review at 45 CFR 46 are not applicable to research involving alternative medicine.

   b. Research involving alternative medicine should be done in full compliance with federal regulations at 45 CFR 46.

   c. It is not ethical to conduct research involving alternative medicine.

   d. The National Institutes of Health will not fund research involving alternative medicine.

3. Choose the most accurate statement:

   a. Complementary and alternative medicine (CAM) medical practices are well-defined and homogenous.

   b. Most CAM practices are easily explained by the Western biomedical model.

   c. Most CAM practices originated in America.

   d. Most CAM practices do not easily fit into the Western biomedical model.

4. Who should provide necessary information about the purity and consistency of an herbal product being considered for investigation?

   a. The IRB committee chairperson

   b. The FDA

   c. The principal investigator

   d. The IRB member who has the concern

ANSWER KEY FOR PART 10

Answer Key: Chapter 10-1

1. b
2. c
3. c

Answer Key: Chapter 10-2

1. c
2. a
3. b

Answer Key: Chapter 10-3

1. c
2. d
3. b
4. a
5. c

Answer Key: Chapter 10-4

1. d
2. b
3. b
4. c
5. b

Answer Key: Chapter 10-5

1. d
2. b
3. a

Answer Key: Chapter 10-6

1. a
2. b
3. b
4. a

Answer Key: Chapter 10-7

1. b
2. a
3. c
4. b

Answer Key: Chapter 10-8

1. c
2. b
3. b
4. a
5. b

Answer Key: Chapter 10-9

1. b
2. d

Answer Key: Chapter 10-10

1. b
2. a
3. c
4. c

Answer Key: Chapter 10-11

1. c
2. b
3. c
4. d

Answer Key: Chapter 10-12

1. b
2. c
3. a
4. d
5. c
6. b

Answer Key: Chapter 10-13

1. a
2. c
3. b
4. d
5. a

Answer Key: Chapter 10-14

1. a
2. a
3. a

Answer Key: Chapter 10-15

1. a
2. b
3. c
4. c

Answer Key: Chapter 10-16

1. d
2. b
3. d
4. c

Part 11

Reference Material and Contact Information

Chapter 11-1B

The Belmont Report

1. *The Belmont Report*

   a. Is now federal law

   b. Explains the policy of the Department of Health and Human Services regarding international research

   c. Was written by representatives of the Food and Drug Administration

   d. Identifies the basic ethical principles that should underlie the conduct of biomedical and behavioral research involving human subjects

2. Choose the answer that most accurately summarizes a statement from Part A (Boundaries Between Research and Practice) of *The Belmont Report*:

   a. The term "practice" refers to interventions that are designed solely to enhance the well-being of an individual patient or client and that have a reasonable expectation of success.

   b. Publication of results in an academic journal defines an activity as research.

   c. A project that involves scientific methodology, such as statistical comparisons, should be considered research from the regulatory standpoint.

   d. When a clinician departs in a significant way from standard or accepted practice, the innovation always constitutes research.

3. Three basic ethical principles described in *The Belmont Report* are

   a. Respect for persons, beneficence, justice

   b. Respect for persons, veracity, justice

   c. Advance society, beneficence, justice

   d. Respect for persons, beneficence, truthfulness

4. Choose the statement that most accurately describes *The Belmont Report's* concept of respect for persons:

   a. Do unto others as you would have them do unto you.

   b. Investigators should direct subjects to make the right decision.

   c. Treat all subjects as autonomous agents with the right to control their own destiny.

   d. Promote truth and honesty when discussing research with potential subjects.

5. Choose the statement that most accurately describes *The Belmont Report's* concept of beneficence:

   a. Distribute the benefits and burdens of research equitably.

   b. Do not act in a way that is likely to cause harm.

   c. Treat all subjects as autonomous agents with the right to control their own destiny.

   d. Do more than "do no harm." Act to maximize potential benefits and minimize potential harms.

6. Choose the statement that most accurately describes *The Belmont Report's* concept of justice:

   a. Give every subject the correct information.

   b. Distribute the benefits and burdens of research equitably.

   c. Act to maximize potential benefits and minimize potential harms.

   d. Treat all subjects as autonomous agents with the right to control their own destiny.

Chapter 11–1C

World Medical Association Declaration of Helsinki

1. Choose the answer that most accurately summarizes a point made in one of the 32 declarations listed in this document:

   a. Individuals have a moral obligation to participate in research that benefits society.

   b. The primary obligation of the physician–researcher is to promote the advancement of science.

   c. In medical research on human subjects, considerations related to the well-being of the human subject should take precedence over the interests of science and society.

   d. Research subjects should ask not what the research will do for them but, rather, what their participation in research will do to benefit society.

2. Choose the answer that most accurately summarizes a point made in one of the 32 declarations listed in this document:

   a. The role of the local investigator is to forward requests for monitoring information to independent committees.

   b. Each local ethical-review committee should duplicate the role of an independent data monitoring board.

   c. The researcher has the obligation to provide monitoring information to the (ethical-review) committee, especially any serious adverse events.

   d. In multisite trials, each local ethical-review committee has the obligation to review every adverse event that is reported at any study site.

3. Choose the answer that most accurately summarizes a point made in one of the 32 declarations listed in this document:

   a. Medical research involving human subjects should be conducted only if the importance of the objective outweighs the inherent risks and burdens to the subject.

   b. Medical research involving human subjects is justified whenever there is the potential that the results of the research will benefit society.

   c. Medical research involving human subjects is justified whenever the risk to subjects in no more than minimal.

   d. Medical research involving human subjects is justified whenever the research is required by the Food and Drug Administration.

4. Choose the answer that most accurately summarizes a point made in one of the 32 declarations listed in this document:

   a. The researcher has the obligation to support the "Therapeutic Misconception" because a positive attitude is likely to improve the health outcome.

   b. It is the responsibility of the subject to be aware of the bias that may exist in discussions with physician–researchers.

   c. Each subject should take a "buyer beware attitude" to participation in research.

   d. If the subject is in a dependent relationship with the physician or may consent under duress, informed consent should be obtained by a well-informed physician who is not engaged in the investigation and who is completely independent of this relationship.

5. Choose the answer that most accurately summarizes a point made in one of the 32 declarations listed in this document:

   a. The study sponsor has the right to control how results will be analyzed and presented.

   b. Care should be taken to avoid the publication of negative results, as this may discourage important research in the future.

   c. After a study has been completed, the study sponsor is entitled to decide whether the results should be published.

   d. In publication of research results, the investigators are obliged to preserve the accuracy of the results. Negative as well as positive results should be published or otherwise publicly made available.

6. Choose the answer that most accurately summarizes a point made in one of the 32 declarations listed in this document:

   a. The policies and procedures to protect the rights and welfare of patients should be identical for medical care and medical research.

   b. When medical research is combined with medical care, additional standards apply to protect the patients who are research subjects.

   c. When medical research is combined with medical care, informed consent for one activity means that there is informed consent for both activities.

   d. Medical research should never be combined with medical care.

7. Choose the answer that most accurately summarizes a point made in one of the 32 declarations listed in this document:

   a. Placebo-controlled trials are required whenever there is doubt about the efficacy of a new medication.

   b. It is never justified to use placebo treatments in medical research.

   c. The benefits, risks, burdens, and effectiveness of a new method should be tested against those of the best current prophylactic, diagnostic, and therapeutic methods.

   d. Placebo-controlled trials are required whenever the active control trial would require a large number of subjects.

ANSWER KEY FOR PART 11

Answer Key: Chapter 11–1B

1. d
2. a
3. a
4. c
5. d
6. b

Answer Key: Chapter 11–1C

1. c
2. c
3. a
4. d
5. d
6. b
7. c